COHERENCE
Revolution

Finding flow on your journey to the present moment

First published in Canada in 2021

www.thecoherencerevolution.com
www.coherencerevolution.com

Cover design by Nailia Minnebaeva
Book interior design by Yuliya Tretyak

This book is intended as a reference volume only, not as a medical manual.

The information given here is designed to help you make informed decisions about your health. It is not intended as a substitute for any treatment that may have been prescribed by your doctor. Neither the publisher nor the author is engaged in rendering professional advice. The ideas, procedures and suggestions, contained in this book are not intended as a substitute for consulting with your physician. Neither the author nor publisher shall be liable or responsible for any loss or damage allegedly arising from any information or suggestion in this book.

Mention of specific companies, organizations or authorities in this book does not imply endorsement by the author or publisher, nor does mention of specific companies, organizations or authorities imply that they endorse this book, its author or the publisher. Internet addresses and telephone numbers given in this book were accurate at the time it went to press.

HeartMath is a registered trademark of Quantum Intech, Inc. For all HeartMath trademarks go to www.heartmath.com/trademarks.

Printed in Canada and the United States of America

Publisher's Cataloguing-in-Publication data:
Coherence Revolution: Finding flow on your journey to the present moment / Dr. Mark Halpern
(Book Category: Self-help)

ISBN 978-1-7775408-2-1 E-book
ISBN 978-1-7775408-1-4 Hardback
ISBN 978-1-7775408-0-7 Paperback

I'd like to dedicate this book to the three most important people in my life.

I am forever grateful for the love and support of my wife, Aviva, who has been an integral part of every aspect of **Coherence Revolution.** Whether it was editing and brainstorming together, or simply lifting me up when necessary, she was a true partner throughout the whole process. I am constantly in awe of the depth of her empathy and love for those around her.

I would also like to dedicate this book to my two kids, Jessica and Andrew. They inspire me to keep going during difficult times and remind me of the simple joys in life. One of the biggest joys and pleasures in my life is having the opportunity to help guide them and watch them grow into the unique and special people they are.

CONTENTS

FOREWORD

You've no doubt sat through a meeting or two and watched a presentation crash and burn, thinking to yourself, 'What an incoherent presentation that was!' Or maybe you saw somebody mumbling and staggering out of a bar late at night and said to your friend, 'That guy is totally incoherent.' Or you listened to a politician inventing words or making no sense whatsoever, and angrily said, 'What an incoherent fool!'

Notice how we refer to all these scenarios as *incoherent*.

Even if you don't know the definition of incoherent, you've figured out it's used to mean sub-par, confused or worse.

If you studied physics in high school or college (and were able to stay awake through it!) you would have learned about the importance of coherence in wave forms, such as light or sound.

Lasers create what physicists call *coherent light,* since the waves and particles emitted by the laser are completely ordered and in sync, flowing in a defined, consistent, predictable pattern.

On the other hand, regular light sources such as incandescent, fluorescent or LED lights are defined by physics as emitting *incoherent light* since the light waves and particles are not aligned and ordered. Instead, they bounce off each other. They do a great job of generally illuminating a room or a space but there's not much precision.

Lasers are capable of incredible precision and effectiveness due to their high degree of order, or coherence. They can scan bar codes; they can shine tiny beams of red light way across a large room during presentations. Sophisticated lasers can surgically repair a retina or knee cartilage, and a host of other remarkable feats. Their exceedingly high degree of order, or coherence, at very low power is their secret.

Try repairing a retina with a 60-watt bulb from Home Depot. Not gonna happen. (Do not try this at home!)

In the early 1990s I was part of the founding leadership team of The HeartMath® Institute, one of the greatest honors of my life. I would frequently co-deliver the introductory science presentation with our research director, Dr. Rollin McCraty. Part of each presentation included the analogy of the laser's coherent light as it was so appropriate for how the human system works.

Most humans are just getting by in life, like a regular light bulb that does a fine job keeping the kitchen bright but eventually burns out. We can get by for a while on innate skills and capacities, but many people are not operating anywhere near their full potential. To put it in this context, most of us are not exactly lasers, producing exceptional precision and power at remarkably low power.

In those early HeartMath days, we asked ourselves, *What if people could be taught to train their systems to be more like a laser – ordered, efficient, precise and coherent – and less like a lamp light, unfocused, overheated and prone to burning out?*

As we began studying the physiology of the heart, particularly as we began doing in-depth research utilizing Heart Rate Variability, we began to realize that the rhythms of the human heart itself follow these same rules of physics as does light.

We discovered that when someone is experiencing a depleting stressful emotion, the heart's rhythmic pattern is actually disordered, unpredictable and incoherent. More energy is required by the heart when

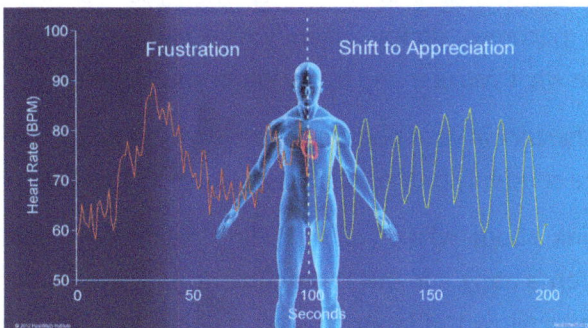

Image courtesy of the HeartMath® Institute – www.heartmath.org

we're in a stress state since our system is incoherent and not efficient, so we tire out more easily.

But our research also uncovered that when people experience positive renewing emotions such as gratitude, love, humor, compassion or peace, the rhythms of their heart become extremely ordered, smooth and efficient. You are saving energy while your system is being restored.

Think about it from your own life experience. When you're stressed out, it can be very draining! Your insides feel chaotic sometimes, certainly not ordered, smooth and efficient. But when you're feeling positive emotionally, it's energizing. Your perspectives are more positive and your energy is much higher.

Positivity is not draining; negativity is. Positivity is energy-producing; negativity is not.

Studying heart rate variability showed us a simple explanation of why.

When you're in a stressful state, it's because something is happening in your life – or you're *afraid* something might happen – that's not what you want. That internal conflict – worry, frustration or anger – causes the rhythms of your heart to become irregular and incoherent. Your body is spending a lot of energy to stay frustrated, which is why you're also so exhausted after a particularly stressful experience. Not only is your heart experiencing the effects of stress, those moment by moment heart beats beating chaotically get circulated all through the body, including your brain! Ever wondered why your IQ seems to drop 30-40 points when you're angry, or why your coordination becomes sloppy when you're rushing, or why you can't communicate what you're trying to say when you're defensive?

The *incoherence* in your body causes every system to go slightly out of sync so you're suddenly only a fraction of who you could be.

Now think about when you're feeling grateful for something – a sunrise, a kitten, a baby, a friend's compliment, your health. We discovered that such times allow the heart to start beating in a beautiful, ordered, energy-efficient and *coherent* rhythm.

In those early years at HeartMath, we also discovered you can easily learn to switch out of the stressful, draining incoherent state into a more efficient, fun and energizing coherent state.

*****

When friends of mine around the world heard I was working with Dr. Mark Halpern and his wife, Aviva Komlos, on a new project called the *Coherence Revolution*, my friends' general reaction was, 'Of course, you are.' The practice and teaching of coherence has been part of my life personally and professionally for thirty years.

Every day I do practices to help me get into a coherent state, help me stay there or help me get back to it when my reaction to stress has pulled me out. Mark has outlined these practices and many more in this marvelous and highly practical book.

A little more than ten years ago my ability to stay coherent was severely challenged when I received a diagnosis of cancer, which required surgery to remove the large tumor and immunotherapy treatments to assure it wouldn't return. The following 18 months were harrowing to be sure, and included repeat staph infections which eventually resulted in a diagnosis of life-threatening MRSA, a particularly hard to treat version of staph which was floating around in my blood.

When some people hear this story they think, 'Guess all that coherence stuff isn't what it's cracked up to be if you got cancer.' And my response is always, 'I never said being coherent will cure all ills or prevent anything bad from ever happening. But I will also say that being coherent mentally, emotionally, physically and spiritually gives yourself the best shot at maximizing your self-healing power.'

Which is exactly what happened to me.

As I write this almost 11 years to the day since my cancer surgery, I can say with all humility that my health is the strongest it's been in decades, thanks in large part to my ongoing commitment to practicing *coherence*. I have weathered deaths in my family, the loss of my marriage, the passing of my mother, several life reinventions, moving from the Bay Area back to New York City and changing careers mid-pandemic.

Now I live life as fully, lovingly, gratefully and as coherently as possible.

My goal – and the goal of this book – is not that you should lead a 100% coherent life. That would be idealistic and unreachable. And always frustrating (and therefore, incoherent!). My goal is to be as coherent as I can be in every situation I'm in so I can be as loving, as thoughtful, as authentic, as wise, as helpful, as supportive, as energizing, as inspiring, as clear, as vulnerable and as compassionate as I can be.

I know that learning, practicing and applying the tools to create coherence that are outlined so masterfully in the pages to come, can become a gentle yet profound revolution in your life.

Welcome to this fantastic journey!

Bruce Cryer
November 2020
Southington, Connecticut

PREFACE

You never change things by fighting the existing reality.
To change something, build a new model that makes
the existing model obsolete.
*— **Buckminster Fuller***

Why is a revolution necessary?

When COVID-19 forced the world to shut down many of us realised just how badly we needed a pause. People's lives were spinning out of control.

I spoke with family, friends and patients who were facing mounting uncertainties, anxieties and overwhelming stress.

The time had come for me to use my life journey, all of my experiences, my setbacks and challenges, my triumphs and healings. It was time to create meaning out of it all. It was time to support others, encourage, inspire and create a pathway that others could follow. It was time for the *Coherence Revolution*.

The fact is most of us work too hard for too many hours.

Disease is increasing at exponential rates no matter how many charities raise money or how many scientists create new medications and treatments.

Animal species are becoming extinct. The ozone is sick and global warming is reaching the point of no return.

We spend more and more of our time on screens and technology, and we are losing our ability to connect with other people.

The world is in need of repair and healing.

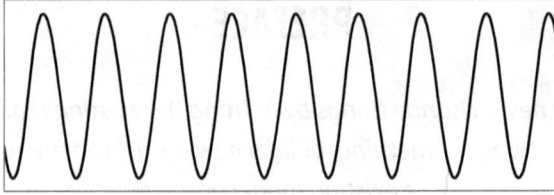

Coherent Sine Wave

Overwhelming choices and the never-ending search

We live in an interesting time. There has never been more information available at our fingertips. You can google and learn about any topic you want and have an answer in only a few seconds. There is an exhaustive amount of information from endless sources.

When it comes to googling and searching for information about various health concerns, it becomes both a blessing and a curse. There is just so much information and many variables to take into account. Does the solution address your need? What are all the choices? What is your philosophy and understanding of the issue? Is there reputable research on it? Who is the source? Do they have a bias? How do you know? Are there other options? How much is it? Is it accessible and available? Who else uses it and recommends it? What are the side effects and dangers? Should I read and pay attention to the comments and reviews? Is what I am learning true?

What you begin to realize is that there are many perceptions of the truth.

The reality of our current healthcare system is that it is based upon outdated laws and scientific theories that are being questioned or adapted as a result of ongoing research.

Ultimately, we each have to decide what makes sense to us and how proactive we choose to be about getting help from those who can guide us.

My search to alleviate the symptoms of stress and anxiety started almost 30 years ago. One of my biggest challenges has always been filtering through the overwhelming number of choices and opinions about health and healing.

For most people, it is challenging to decide the best course of action because they start their search when they are already suffering. A sense of desperation is created to find answers.

It took me many years to change my attitude from one of desperation to one of inspiration. By focusing on the process of creating coherence, I reconnected with my sense of self, my core being and my heart. I raised my frequency.

I became a curious co-creator of my life when I learned the tools and developed a process to follow. I learned to listen to the whisperings of my heart and consciously chose to meet each day with increased ease and gratitude.

Why call it the *Coherence Revolution*?

The human body consists of many different physiological systems – each with their own rhythm. To function at an optimal level, each of those systems must resonate and be in tune with the others. The strongest rhythm, and therefore the one that sets the tone for all the others, is the heart rhythm.

Thanks to the pioneering research done by the HeartMath Institute, the term *coherence* has become widely known and associated with emotional health. Over the last 30-plus years, HeartMath has developed and taught the concept of heart / brain coherence. One of their first and still most profound discoveries was that the visual representation of a Coherent Heart rhythm is a perfect sine wave.

Every time I think about or talk about the *Coherence Revolution*, I visualize a sine wave and feel the flow of the wave. Simply thinking about coherence increases it. When I think about coherence, I think of rhythm. I think of balance. I think of being in tune with myself and with the world around me.

To me, *revolution* is about seeking drastic change by creating a fundamentally new way of being. It represents people coming together with a common purpose or cause.

That is exactly what this program is all about.

The *Coherence Revolution* is for seekers who want more from life and are willing to put in the effort to get it.

It's for people willing to do the self-inquiry necessary to make real change within.

It's for those who are willing to go outside of their comfort zone.

It's for people who are open to being curious, creative, silly and childlike.

It's for people who love themselves enough to create the best life they possibly can.

And it's for people who understand that the quality of the life they lead influences the lives of everyone else on the planet.

Who would benefit from reading this book?

There are thousands of books and authors who deliver similar messages of growth through adversity and change as an outcome from chaos. In most cases, it is not just the message that is attractive; it's who delivers it, their unique story and how they present it so that it becomes relevant for your life.

Throughout my journey, I've always found little gems that changed my life forever. Whether it was a self-help program, a CD box set, a seminar, a book or a specific therapist, I am forever grateful that I have had the opportunity to learn and implement so many impactful concepts and tools.

In developing the *Coherence Revolution*, I built upon concepts from some of the most influential books I've read and programs I've taken.

I focus on the aspects I believe are the most accessible to the greatest amount of people.

If you are interested to learn more about any of the programs, books or people I mention, I encourage you to do so. My intention is to interpret the information in such a way that the concept of coherence is understandable and attainable for anyone who puts in the effort to make a change.

I take the responsibility of sharing this information seriously and am grateful for the opportunity to guide people through their journey of creating a coherent life.

I have had many detours with extremely bumpy roads and crashes along the way. For some time I hesitated to write a book because I have not succeeded at eliminating anxiety entirely from my life. I still suffer from time to time. My life is not always composed of rainbows and sunshine. It can be really challenging and frustrating at times.

There are millions of people every day searching. Searching desperately for some*one* or some*thing* to help guide them, to give them some relief, to give them hope, to tell them they are going in the right direction or to prevent them from going down the wrong path.

People are looking for short-term relief but need long-term solutions. It's very confusing.

So, what can you do? Who can help?

If you are like me, you want *simple answers* that are easy to understand and implement.

I believe that the more information people have, the better decisions they can make. I don't want to discourage you from being thorough. I want to help you avoid all the endless searching.

My tendency, during my seemingly endless search for answers, was to approach anxiety from every single angle and perspective until I found the answer that was going to change my life.

I saw kidney specialists and adrenal specialists, had food sensitivity testing, wore a heart monitor and had every system in my body evaluated. In my case, as with the majority of people, none of that testing resulted in any change to my health or gave me hope for the future.

I have gone through more typical approaches to anxiety such as medication, psychotherapy, self-help books and cognitive behavioral approaches. I have also explored a plethora of alternative methods and approaches that many people would find hard to believe and would never even consider trying.

I have experienced the frustration that comes with a vague or oversimplified diagnosis. I have encountered practitioners who believed they had *figured me* out and promised I would feel better in a short period of time.

I understand what it's like to be told that things will get better in time – endless amounts of time. I was told, 'It will take time,' over and over and over. If one more person told me they could help, I was going to scream! I wanted to heal *now*.

I recall one specific session with an Energy practitioner when I felt particularly desperate for answers. At the time, she told me that I would eventually heal, but it would take another year and a half to feel some relief. This felt like a death sentence. I didn't want to wait another day, let alone a year and a half. In that moment, I felt a surge of uncertainty and doubt. I desperately didn't want to wait that long. How could I continue to wake up every day and experience anxiety? How could I get through the financial strain I was feeling? How could I still be a good husband and father?

I just didn't want to wait to get 'there.' 'There' was a place where I could handle anxiety without medication, a place where I felt good and a place where I had enough money to live our chosen lifestyle. I was always desperate to get 'there.'

It's now been five years since that appointment and I am still not 'there.' I continued to work, earned enough money to pay the bills, went on a few vacations and made sure the kids had everything they could possibly need. I have continued to take courses, build my practice and learn as much as I can about all my passions. I have dealt with health concerns, gone on and off medication and created plenty of good habits. I am still not 'there.'

It took me a long time to figure this out, but there is no 'there.'

Life is about the *process,* not the *destination*. It seems like most people are waiting to be happy or healthy until they have reached their goal or completed their course, got married, made enough money, went on vacation or got the new job.

This is my life. There is nothing to wait for. I have chosen very specific daily habits, rituals and activities to engage in with the intention of creating and living my dream life.

As John Lennon said, 'Life is what happens while you're busy making other plans.'

Section 1

MY JOURNEY

Chapter 1

THE PAUSE

And just like that, life was paused. It didn't require months of planning. There were no difficult logistics. I just closed my office, picked up a few groceries and headed home. On break. Pause. Indefinite hold. Just about every aspect of my life was instantly thrust into uncertainty.

Every trigger and insecurity I've struggled with bubbled to the surface. How long will this go on? How long can we afford to live our lifestyle? Will I have to completely rebuild? I wasn't even sure if co-parenting would work. Could my kids continue living in two homes?

Each of these issues had the potential power to trigger a massive response. My typical process usually included severe anxiety and emotional instability. But it didn't happen. There was almost a calm that came over me. It was a relief.

A realization came over me that had I not been forced to take the time to heal, I would never have taken enough time off to truly heal in all areas of my life. I saw this forced layoff for what it truly was. *A gift.* When else was I going to get the opportunity to take a break from *regular life* for at least three months?

I was acutely aware that I had done a lot of work over many years in preparation for this type of situation. When all of it hit at once, I knew it was epic. I knew it was scary. I knew it was going to be very impactful. But terror did not strike. Even with all that was going on, I knew I had tools and I also knew how good this time would be for my family and me. I could not imagine more uncertainty or unknown. And yet, I was excited. I saw an opportunity. There couldn't possibly be a better time for the creation of the *Coherence Revolution*!

I've thought about writing 'my book' for 20 years. Initially, I made jokes with friends and even therapists about the book I should write, as I felt that my life had become quite intense and dramatic. I may have only been in my twenties but all of the anxiety programs and visits to therapists had begun to pile up.

Speaking about writing a book was almost like paying homage to how difficult my journey had been. It signified relevance and importance. It gave meaning to my suffering. Over time, though, the idea of writing a book became more serious. I knew that my accomplishments, and even mishaps, could inspire others. I knew that my extreme focus on self-care and searching for answers to help with anxiety could help change other people's lives as well as my own. I knew that I could help others in their search. I could make it easier. I could help them avoid the same roadblocks.

My hesitation has always been that I am not *ALL BETTER*.

I am not free of anxiety. I still get emotional. At times, life can still feel like a struggle.

What is ALL BETTER? We are never a final product. I always thought I'd find the answer to my problems and fix them. I felt that only then, I could be someone people would believe and trust. I believed I was an imposter or a fraud. I didn't think anyone could look up to me or respect me if they knew what was really going on inside.

As I shifted my focus from problem solving to creating more flow and balance, life became simpler. My focus, intentions and goals became clearer to me.

Creating coherence does not mean you don't have problems or that issues won't arise in the future. It means that you have many tools at your disposal, which you can use to support yourself through challenging times. It means that you have a better understanding of what fuels you or calms you so that each moment is less draining. It means that you connect with awareness and resilience. It means you have a much better chance for success. Coherence lessens the state of stress within.

Coherence is not about making more money, but it can lead to that. Coherence is about creating a coherent lifestyle within your financial means. It's not about needing friends, family or a spouse. It's about surrounding yourself with people you feel in coherence with and who bring out the best in you so you have a community that is vibrant, nurturing and inspiring.

When you focus on creating more coherence in the moment, it helps shift your thoughts away from getting rid of specific symptoms, solving stressful situations or resolving emotional disputes.

The intention, in the moment, is to create as much coherence as possible in every cell, tissue and organ system so they will function optimally, respond appropriately and be able to adapt to their environment.

Like health, *coherence* is a state of being rather than a place or a thing. Ideally, your body, mind and spirit are always operating in a healthy state.

The same can also be said of happiness. People talk about their search for happiness. But it's not a search; it's a practice.

If you consistently practice being healthy and happy every day, it will transform your life into one of joy, passion, inspiration and true coherence.

Chapter 2

MY BEGINNING

After innumerable initial consultations with different practitioners and therapists, I could review and tell my story in my sleep. It's amazing how succinct you can become when describing your life.

As upbringings go, mine was great. I was surrounded by a lot of love and support. My parents and I often joke that none of us remember the details of my early childhood such as bedtime cuddles, story time or playing games together but we all share the same sense of love and warmth in our memories. That time of my life feels so innocent and pure.

My mom and dad were always there with a supportive comment and encouragement. They made sure I ate well, slept well and that I was always involved with a wide variety of activities. They helped me with schoolwork, talked through difficulties and challenges, and gave me the freedom to play and be a child.

I was pretty much raised in a middle-class family. We didn't have a lot of extra money, but my parents sacrificed so I could have what I needed and could continue to do the things I loved. Even when we didn't have a ton of money, they would always find a way for me to get at least one of the trendy items that were 'in.' Whether it was an extra-curricular program, a new jacket, bike or piece of jewelry, my parents always found a way to make sure I wasn't left out.

I would say I was a social child and I always seemed to have many friends in my life. For the most part, I was a popular kid at school. I was both a bully and the bullied. Both existed and sometimes on the same day. It seemed like there was always a hierarchy in the schoolyard. There were the perceived groups of 'cool kids,' 'losers' and 'nerds.' On any given day, the group you 'fit into' was dependent on who was making the judgment. Peer pressure, ego and insecurity were pretty powerful influences on my sense of self.

I had several features that were ripe for people to pick on – thick glasses, curly hair and being short were the most obvious targets. They all caused me to feel even worse about myself. So being an equal-opportunity person, I teased kids who I perceived to be even lower on the hierarchy system than I was. I always had a good heart, but at the time it was easy to take my frustrations out on people I believed were easy targets.

As a child, I would play or engage in just about any sport or activity that I was introduced to including hockey, baseball, soccer, BMX biking, mountain biking, roller blading, billiards, sailing, swimming, skiing, water skiing, golf, frisbee, volleyball, camping, gaga, tether ball, football, tag and even red rover.

Sleepover camp in the summer was a really special place for me. There was no place on earth where I had more confidence than summer camp. It just felt right to be there and I felt accepted. Talk about feeling coherent in your surroundings! To this day, when I visit my kids at the same camp I went to, I still feel the emotions I felt as a child when I walk around the grounds.

Until the end of grade six I felt confident, had friends and there was definitely nothing that would have concerned my parents, teachers or any adult who spent time with me. I wasn't the child who threw tantrums. I wasn't excessively stubborn. I wasn't angry. I wasn't an anxious child at all. From an emotional perspective, my life felt as though it was unfolding smoothly. There was nothing that would have alerted anyone, including myself, that I was a child about to develop terrible insecurities.

The transition from grade six to seven was a pivotal time for me. That's probably pretty typical timing for teenage angst to begin. There were certainly many natural changes occurring internally and externally that made it even more challenging to make the jump to junior high school. During those years, my self-esteem began to diminish and I tried desperately to be liked and accepted.

On the surface, it looked like I was popular with a big group of friends. However, internally, I was starting to feel very insecure around other teenagers. Situations which were once comfortable for me became the grounds for heightened insecurity. I started doubting myself and feeling emotions that would eventually affect my behavior. I hadn't experienced severe anxiety yet, but the emotional damage was accumulating and negative emotional responses were already becoming habitual.

It all spiraled down from there. I constantly repeated terrible thinking habits without realizing it. The result was that I started inadvertently practicing what I ultimately became very proficient at, which was my ability to get and stay anxious.

Yes, I became pretty good. And by that I mean, I excelled in my ability to get anxious. There was no one who could do it better. Unfortunately, I was young and had little awareness of my emotions or that I should reach out for help.

I continued reacting and responding in the same way, and over time, it became a hardwired neurological program. By the time I was into my teen years, an anxiety response could be triggered by just about any teen stressor – socializing, popularity, drugs, alcohol, schooling, etc.

As a teen in the '80s, I was not exposed to open conversations about mental health. It wasn't common to discuss emotions or self-regulation in any meaningful way. I found that most kids didn't know how to cope with a friend with anxiety. More importantly, I didn't know how to cope with myself.

As a father, I am profoundly grateful that my children are learning how to avoid the same patterns I developed and have a chance to create a completely different life experience.

Chapter 3

PRACTICING ANXIETY

The great thing about hindsight within a coherent mindset is that I truly understand that my health and wellbeing has nothing to do with what people did or didn't do to me or towards me. In every single situation, I had a choice about what to think and how to respond. I just may not have realized it or perhaps did not like my choices.

Taking responsibility is essential. As long as I perceived that my anxiety was the result of someone else's wrongdoing, I couldn't heal. As long as it was the external stress that was to blame for the anxiety I was feeling, I couldn't let it go.

Today, accepting personal responsibility doesn't mean I blame myself for developing the anxiety I experienced. It means I have the *ability* and the *responsibility* to change the situation. It means I can heal from the inside out. It means I choose how I live my life from this moment forward.

As a teen though, I did not yet know how to cope or understand the process that was under way. My mind and body continued to solidify the addiction to repetitive incoherent brain patterns that had been developed at a very young age.

These incoherent brain patterns had a direct effect on my physiological state and coloured the way I saw everything and everyone. The result was generally an increased heart rate, elevated blood pressure and the creation of more stress chemicals that resulted in feelings of fear.

One could say I *practiced* anxiety so much that it became extremely easy to trigger a stress response. On the outside, I appeared fine. But on the inside, my mind was racing, and all the sensations associated with anxiety were becoming my normal state. I constantly experienced symptoms that caused me to feel emotionally unbalanced and frequently had that feeling of nervousness in the pit of my stomach, as if something really scary or terrible was about to happen. It was frustrating for me that I was not receiving the external validation I was seeking while I was in that anxious state. I wanted to be understood, to be liked and to be respected. I wanted to be told that I'd be okay. I essentially wanted to be validated as a human being.

As I look back, I realize that so many of my insecurities, and lack of self-esteem, stemmed from my perception of just a few incidents during my early teen years. To this day, if I choose to relive some of those moments, I can feel the same emotions all over again.

I only remember a few interactions or specific conversations from those very formative years. This is true for most people. As humans, we generally don't remember full details of past conversations. We remember a few words or the gist of what was said, but it's really the tone or the emotions that are felt in that moment. We remember through emotional experience.

In my case, my perceptions of the actions or non-actions of just a few people and a couple of circumstances became ingrained and imprinted in my subconscious. My recollection of the events didn't have to be perfect. All it took to feel the emotions from those events were just a few vague details.

All of us have experienced this at one time or another. When you remember a past event, if there is a strong enough emotion tied to it, you will feel the emotion again simply by remembering the event.

When you are thinking about it and your body is feeling it, your brain isn't going to distinguish whether the event already happened or if it's happening in the present moment. It doesn't matter anymore. The response is hardwired and every time you relive it, the brain is interpreting it as if it's happening again. I've spent close to 40 years trying to undo the damage I allowed to happen during such a significant time in the development of my emotional self-regulation.

I was far more aware than the average teenager about how we communicated with each other. I believe it was due to the fact I was often in a heightened, anxious state. I also watched how people treated each other. I became very adept at reading situations. For the most part, other teenagers I knew didn't seem conscious of how their behavior, their words or their actions might affect others.

Awareness wasn't enough though. I had no idea how to avoid the destructive mental process I was engaged in and I didn't realize I had choices. I allowed the hardwiring process to continue.

As an adult going through the healing process, it was important to avoid blaming myself for allowing the insecurities to develop. It was also very important not to blame others. The healing process couldn't even start until I took full responsibility for my life and released all of the blame towards others.

It is all too common for people to continue to feel the same negative emotions in the present moment as they did when the event occurred. No matter what age you are, when you associate a strong emotion with a memory, you will feel that age again. For a brief second you remember the feelings you felt as a child all over again. It is important to understand that in the present moment, if you're reliving old depleting emotions, there is nothing left in the present to feel bad about.

Hindsight being 20/20, I have often wished I could have a conversation with myself as a child and correct the negative patterns before they had a chance to define that period of my life.

As a father, I have not directly taught my kids how to help or support their friends with stress or anxiety issues. However, since they were very young, we have talked about different emotional states, self-regulation and creating coherence in our lives. I am beyond grateful and proud that they have naturally taken different approaches with their friends and are navigating their early teen years in mindful ways.

It seems like situations arise every few weeks that demonstrate to me the benefits of teaching my kids these principles, and I'm reminded of how different their relationships and social interactions are compared to my childhood experience.

There is one particular example that stands out to me. Around the time my son Andrew turned 12, we had a conversation about a friend of his from school who he felt was very insecure. This boy had been at our house for a small birthday party and in a span of two hours had several huge servings of chips and a six-pack of juice boxes. It seemed like a lot, yet it was no big deal for a 12-year-old boy to gorge on snacks at a birthday party. Later that evening Andrew said to me, 'Dad, you know my friend George [not his real name], and how much he was eating at the party?' I said yes. He continued, 'Well, he eats a lot because he is insecure. I asked him if he was insecure and he said yes. I told him he didn't have to be. And we have this thing where we give each other a playful tap on the forehead as a joke. I do it to him all the time. But every time he does it to me, he says sorry like a million times. I told him he doesn't have to. I told him we are good enough friends that he doesn't have to be insecure with me and that we're all good. I don't want him to worry.'

I am extremely proud of my son and his emotional intelligence. I love the level of awareness Andrew showed and that he was able to communicate it.

The conversation between the two children also had the potential of being an impactful moment in his friend's life, and I felt good for him. If you were an insecure child and one of your friends told you that you matter and that you had permission to be yourself, that would be a gift.

I'm definitely not suggesting our kids are responsible for their friends' insecurities, self-esteem or happiness. That being said, there is power in reflecting on how much impact we potentially have on our friends' lives. Imagine, if at a time of uncertainty and insecurity, someone were to tell you unsolicitedly that you were liked, loved and respected. Imagine how that would feel.

Chapter 4

THERAPY AND SELF-CARE

For most of my adult life, anxiety was a constant. Wherever I went, and whatever I did, there I was. It seemed like the more desperate I was to stop suffering, the worse it got. I never gave up though. There was always something new to give me hope. I started to explore new methods, therapies and diets, and was open to just about any Eastern or Western-based approach to healing as well as any other intriguing alternative I could find. My intention was always to create the best life possible.

I was willing to commit as much time, money and effort as it took to get healthy. When it came to my healing and finding a way to function in our society, I never used finances as an excuse. I always thought of it as an investment in myself and a necessity of life.

I didn't realize how accurate that thought was, seeing as all of those experiences were essentially preparing me to create the *Coherence Revolution*.

Some would say, sarcastically I might add, that I did my research well. I drove an hour and a half to have my saliva checked for heavy metals. During another period of time, I drove over an hour several times per week to try a wand that had zero point energy. I went to a shaman who pulled swords out of my back from wars I fought hundreds of years ago. I sat in practitioners' offices for hours and learned about angels, helpers, guardians and energy blocks. I've carried and displayed crystals. I've tried bodywork, tapping, EFT, Gestalt therapy, Quantum K and The Work (Byron Katie). I participated in dozens of sessions of neurofeedback. I took a Tony Robbins relationship course and have completed several financial mastery seminars. The list goes on. I was fascinated by energy healers, quantum physics, neurophysiology and any other techniques which facilitated healing.

In my late thirties, I had a particularly unusual experience that at the time seemed so normal to me. During that period it felt like my life was unravelling a little bit so I went to a highly recommended channeler, Bart Smit. During the session, Bart channeled his other personality and consciousness, Dr. Williams. His head tilted back and his eyes were closed the entire time after he made the transformation from one consciousness to the other.

We had a very meaningful conversation and he told me he believed that I was having a Kundalini awakening. He explained it could be a long and potentially painful process but that I would be completely transformed over the next several years. He spent quite a bit of time explaining how this awakening applied to the circumstances in my life.

It all made sense. He answered some very practical questions about the past, present and future. It was a surreal circumstance. Oddly, I had no problem ignoring the fact that Bart sat in his chair with his head tilted back and his eyes closed. I remember thinking how trustworthy Dr. Williams seemed.

My first program

In general, I seem to have a hard time recalling the exact age I was for many important events in my life. Around the time I finished high school, stress and mood issues became more serious. I experienced severe anxiety on a daily basis. I remember being confused and trying to understand what anxiety was and why it was affecting me. I became concerned and wanted to be proactive so I could learn how to eliminate it.

Around that time, I read about a program for people suffering with anxiety. The company happened to be giving a free seminar, so I signed up. Although I had never had any meaningful discussions about anxiety with my parents, this was my opportunity to bring them into my world a little bit and share my concerns with them. I asked if they would join me and they accepted without hesitation.

I don't think my parents knew what to make of it all. They came from a generation of people who did not talk about anxiety, although they both, at one time or another, disclosed that they had tendencies that led to overthinking. I think they were happy I was being proactive and were also open to see if it could help them too.

The three of us went and sat through a fairly long, eye-opening lecture. I resonated with enough of the information that I bought the program. It became the first program or treatment of any kind that I engaged in to address and hopefully ease my anxiety. The program was a mixture of CBT (Cognitive Behavioral Therapy) and written exercises to help reframe and reprogram thoughts to help eliminate anxiety.

Looking back, I realize how naive I was. I dove in, did the work, wrote out my assignments and had hope. Like most things I've done since then, I was pretty disappointed when I realized it was not the magic pill to get rid of all the anxiety I was experiencing.

I often wonder what the outcome might have been had I practiced, committed and engaged in the course even more. Interestingly, that first program taught me some of the most important concepts, but I wasn't ready to hear them or fully grasp them yet. Lessons learned and messages received, can and will be interpreted differently depending on the time and your readiness to hear them.

I did learn a lot from that first program even though I was only able to digest the information on a superficial level. It was a really important milestone and I began seeing one of many therapists shortly afterwards.

Going to so many therapists was quite a ride. I went to therapists who laughed at me because I was overly introspective. I was told that I thought too much. I was told to relax more. I was told to reduce my stress level. I've had rude therapists, weird therapists and mystical therapists. I was open to anyone who I thought could help me get rid of anxiety.

Although my experiences varied greatly between practitioners, talk therapy actually accomplished several things for me. It served as an effective means for catharsis, it continued pointing me in a positive direction and it offered hope.

I especially enjoyed the cathartic aspect of therapy, being in someone's office and having permission to purge my emotions. Due to the fact I started therapy with so many different people, I became very good at summarizing my life story. I felt as if I had to catch them up on where I was in my journey so I could pick up where I left off from the last therapist and resume the catharsis.

Most of the therapists I saw would empathize and offer suggestions, but mostly, they just listened. I became an expert at analyzing myself and was able to communicate my experience well. No matter who I saw, I always left feeling a bit better because I had gotten it all out.

Talk therapy does have its limitations though. On many occasions, within minutes of leaving a therapy session, I wanted to go back or at least call a friend so I could continue to go through the issues that were occupying my mind. The cathartic release didn't last long.

After years of therapy, I finally realized that a coherent future will not be the result of simply understanding the past. You can't think yourself or understand yourself out of your past issues.

No matter how well you understand why something happened or how you will respond differently next time, it doesn't eliminate the neural programming that exists. Conscious awareness is a very good thing though. If you know thought patterns and belief systems exist, you have a chance to change, eliminate and rewire them.

Talk therapy is useful to gain some clarity on the aspects of your life that require attention and focus. It's a good first step as part of an overall strategy to gain coherence in every aspect of your life.

Chapter 5

MEDICATIONS AND EXPERIMENTATION

The medication dilemma

I have had a long, confusing and stressful relationship with medications. In general, I believe that medications can be beneficial and potentially lifesaving. When used appropriately, some medications can provide a quality of life for people that otherwise would be unattainable.

My general opposition to medications has evolved over the years. In the past, my biggest concern was regarding drugs with the potential for long-term addiction and the risk of many side effects or dangers. Over the years, as my perception of the world changed, my concerns shifted.

I will always be open to medications that can save and improve the quality of life. However, my concern is that there are too many medications that reduce the body's own ability to self-regulate or create the optimal healing response.

Initially, taking medications didn't bother me at all. As a child, I was vaccinated, my parents gave me pain medications occasionally and I had no problem taking whatever I was given for any ailments or injuries.

During my later childhood, I was prone to headaches and I recall taking Tylenol as far back as grade four or five. By the time I was in my later teen years, I took Tylenol 3s fairly regularly. I wasn't popping pills or abusing pain medication, but I did get frequent headaches, and a couple of regular-strength pills weren't enough to relieve the pain. I remember feeling that I was *cool* because my tolerance for Tylenol was so high. Thankfully, it never became a problem.

On several occasions, I have been prescribed medications to ease my suffering. Although I had different reactions and varied amounts of success with each medication, I felt immense embarrassment and frustration that lasted the entire time I was on it. I constantly ruminated on my perceived weakness for taking it. It bothered me that I had done so much work and still needed the external help.

I felt the image of me having personal struggles with anxiety and taking medications was the exact opposite to my work persona of being the healthy and passionate doctor.

I thought about that a lot. It's a terrible feeling to feel like a fraud. Literally every time I put my hand to my mouth to take the medication (twice per day), I felt guilt, shame and disappointment. Unfortunately, that lasted for many years. Talk about a neurological pattern and trained habit!

I am extremely proud of my transition and growth in this area. Although it is fulfilling and I am truly grateful that I was finally able to eliminate the medication, it was even more satisfying because I had made peace with the use of it before I weaned off. I felt gratitude for the ease it gave me and appreciated the quality of life I achieved during some pretty challenging times. If it weren't for the medication, I would not have been capable of doing all the work and making all the necessary changes in my life.

Experimental years

Growing up, I was considered a good child by almost any standard. I may have been a bit mischievous but in general, I achieved high grades, excelled at sports, had friends and wasn't a cause for concern for either my teachers or my parents.

All of that being true though, I was also a very experimental kid. I enjoyed extreme sports such as BMX biking and skiing, and I enjoyed doing things that were considered risky. I was a bit of a daredevil.

As a teenager, my friends and I were introduced to the music of the Grateful Dead. They were a rock band from the 1960s and founding members of the hippie generation. I could write an entire novel on this phase of my life alone. Between the ages of 16 and 20, my friends and I toured Canada and the United States any chance we got. Typically, my parents let me use their minivan and we hit the road several times per year to go see live music. Depending on the amount of time we had, we would drive just about anywhere. We drove to New Jersey for one show, the Midwest for a weekend, out West for weeks at a time to see dozens of shows, and up and down the East Coast multiple times.

Grateful Dead concerts were unique because every show was different. There were no setlists. If you attended 10 shows, you saw 10 different shows. It was one big party with awesome music, in a circus-like atmosphere. There was nowhere else in the world where you could have that experience. We were a part of a travelling band of hippies.

It was a unique time that most likely couldn't happen today. The world is a different place now. At the time, my parents allowed me to drive their vehicle, with no phone or way to communicate with them other than to find a pay phone. We had several maps with the main highways indicated but very little else. I don't know too many parents today who would let their teenager do that.

Since I was a good student who stayed out of trouble and always took care of my responsibilities, my parents showed faith and trust in me and gave me the freedom to go on those adventures.

The concerts we saw and the tours we took were as much or more about the journey as they were about the music. We were truly free. In between concerts, we'd explore Canada and the U.S. We hiked in the mountains, swam under waterfalls and discovered the spiritual aspects of ourselves. It was a time of great personal discovery and psychedelic experimentation.

Looking back, it blows my mind how young we really were to be on our own and exploring life with no boundaries. It's safe to say, we had a lot of fun and found ourselves in some pretty outrageous situations. I am, however, proud and even a bit relieved that those experiences, in hindsight, were less about partying and more about my journey to self-discovery. I learned a lot of invaluable life lessons.

It would be misleading to say that I enjoyed every minute of it. I didn't, but I do not regret any of my experiences even though some of them happened at potentially sensitive and vulnerable times.

The lens from which I view drugs and medications has never been simple or straightforward. I've never really worried about ingesting over-the-counter drugs, natural medicines or recreational drugs. It was only the prescribed medications I had a problem with. My opposition to taking medications was due more to the shame and guilt I had associated with it than the potential danger of the drugs. My resistance to taking medication had nothing to do with it being natural or unnatural. I simply felt like I was weak and unhealthy if I needed medications. It hurt my ego to feel like something was wrong with me. I felt embarrassed, like I was a fraud.

I also had some philosophical objections to taking medications. I started chiropractic college when I was 20 years old and have been caring for people and teaching holistic principles for close to 25 years. One of the most basic principles I talk about is the body's innate wisdom – our ability to self-regulate and heal. At the most fundamental level, my job is to help facilitate healing from the inside out, not from the outside in.

Thankfully, I didn't let my ego get in the way of trying. My desire to get rid of anxiety was always much stronger than my aversion to medication, so when it was recommended, I considered my options. Although it took me many years, eventually I felt gratitude for the benefits I received.

There were times medications gave me at least some quality of life. There were times I wouldn't have been able to leave the house. I wouldn't have been able to read the books, attend the lectures or go to the workshops. It took me a really long time to stop judging myself and to look at the big picture. There was so much unnecessary self-judgement that only served to make my journey more difficult than it needed to be.

Chapter 6

LEARNING EMOTION THROUGH MUSIC

Travelling and touring to go see the Grateful Dead defined my early adulthood. My childhood friends were becoming my lifelong friends, and the music I was listening to would go on to become the soundtrack of my life. It was a time where I learned to give affection and love to others and a time when I opened my mind to new concepts and perceptions of reality.

The entire Grateful Dead scene was based on a foundation of love. Love for the music, the band and the community. Love for the adventure and love for the exploration and the journey. While it was still many years before being introduced to quantum physics and all of the brilliant people who have changed my life, the Grateful Dead was my first exposure to people loving each other without hesitation or pretense. My friends and I were only 16 but we hugged each other all the time. It was quite a unique way to start learning how to live a heart-centered life.

There are so many concepts that I now teach or have implemented in my life that I can trace back to my experience at Grateful Dead concerts. At the core of the experience was the music, which was soulful and full of emotions. There were moments at just about every concert I saw, when the band was in *the zone* and everyone in the audience was right there with them. We could feel the peak of the music building. It was palpable. It was *coherent*. At times, it felt orgasmic. Time stood still. The musicians were not only connected and in complete flow with each other but also with the audience.

Whether they wanted to get the audience dancing or they wanted to tug at their heartstrings, it was an emotional experience from start to finish. The band strategically chose songs at the appropriate times. And that was why I went back night after night.

A unique fact about the Grateful Dead is that they allowed their fans to tape their shows, and due to the fact they have performed more live shows than any rock band in history, there are recordings of over 2500 shows. I am extremely grateful and amazed that more than 30 years later, I have access to technology that gives me the ability to listen to every concert I went to. I often start listening from the first show I saw and progressively go through each year.

Music is one of the most powerful ways to elicit an emotion, and since the Grateful Dead were particularly masterful at guiding the audience through an emotional journey, sometimes I'll listen to a specific show based upon the emotion I want to relive.

Chapter 7

SPIRITUALITY VS RELIGION VS SCIENCE

I was brought up in a conservative Jewish household. My parents went to synagogue on the holidays and observed some of the basic Jewish traditions. I went to Hebrew school and had a bar mitzvah, as did all of my Jewish friends. I was a good student and did well but I never connected with the religious teachings. I never felt comfortable praying the way it was presented to me. I didn't believe there was an omnipotent god who made decisions and determined what happened in people's lives. I didn't believe there was a being or entity who punished people if they didn't listen or live their life by some random definition of a moral code.

I never looked to religion as a source of positive messages or life lessons because I just wasn't connecting with the religious teachings. My bar mitzvah was really the end of any formal Jewish learning.

The first book I read on spirituality that inspired me was *On the Road* by Jack Kerouac. It was about the *Beatniks* in the pre-hippie days of the late 1950s and early 1960s. I started reading it around the same time I started travelling and seeing the Grateful Dead, so the book really resonated with me.

Shortly after that, I also read *Jonathan Livingston Seagull*. It's a book about a seagull who was different from all the other seagulls. He wanted to fly higher and soar further in his life than the boundaries set forth by the others.

As I reached the end of my teen years and entered my twenties, I was gaining more interest in spiritual concepts. The first time I attempted meditation was in my early twenties. I bought a book by Shakti Gawain called *Creative Visualization*. I remember sitting down to meditate and feeling like I wasn't doing it correctly. I had a hard time getting my mind to shut off. I liked the concept of meditation, but I gave up after a few weeks. Looking back, I realize I wasn't ready to actually start a meditation practice. I was focusing on getting immediate results rather than creating positive habits.

Perhaps the most influential book I read in my early twenties was *The Celestine Prophecy* by James Redfield. Although it was a book of fiction, some of the concepts inspired me. I remember one example from the book that was impactful and I still think about it to this day.

The main character related a principle he was learning with regards to those who come into our lives. He relayed that when you cross paths with someone and your eyes lock, it's an indication that there is something to be communicated between the two of you. It means there is some piece of relevant information or knowledge that is meant to be shared.

I have never forgotten this concept, and every time I meet someone's eyes, I think to myself, *What do they have to tell me?*

It is much easier to sense non-verbal communication when you are feeling coherent within and with your surroundings. If you are inspired and feeling coherent, the chance of you taking action and communicating with that person is much greater. If you are incoherent and not feeling authentically yourself, the opportunity for any exchange is most likely lost.

Whether through a book, course, seminar or teacher, I have been exploring spirituality in all of its forms for close to 30 years. I have held or worn magnets, crystals and stones. I've posted positive affirmations all over my home and workspace and recited them daily. I've asked the Universe, God, the quantum field, angels and any other recommended spiritual beings to give me answers and help me heal.

We are in a fascinating and uniquely powerful time regarding spirituality and science. Science is attempting to prove and delve into some typically philosophical concepts behind spirituality and religion.

It's one thing to be taught that meditation is a great habit to practice as part of a healthy lifestyle. It's a whole other thing to learn the specific parts of the brain that function better and spontaneously heal as a result of meditation.

It's much easier to see why teaching someone to be grateful is a gift once they understand that practicing gratitude can lead to profound healings.

Most religions and spiritual practices teach similar messages and common themes such as love for self, love for others and love for our planet.

Thanks to quantum science and organizations such as HeartMath, there is a growing body of research that shows that the power of love can actually help heal your body, your relationships and the entire planet.

I am greatly inspired by this.

Meditation, energy work, gratitude and opening the heart are all concepts that have become much more accessible and understandable. They aren't abstract anymore. They are real concepts that can be practiced and learned.

What if the secret to life is much simpler than we ever imagined? How great would it be if we realized that the stories passed down for thousands of years by religious leaders were simply teaching us that by practicing and feeling the emotion of love, we can heal our brain and body, our human connections, the ozone and the oceans? There is still much research to be done but we are getting a lot closer to understanding how coherent and renewing emotions impact the health of our species as well as the planet.

Chapter 8

EDUCATED AND STILL STRUGGLING

Unless you were close to me personally, you would never have known the extent of my inner struggles. I was one of the youngest chiropractors in Canada when I graduated. I had drive and ambition. I was willing to take courses, attend seminars, promote my practice, give lectures in the community and generally do whatever it took to be successful.

I took pride in my effort and ability to overcome my fears and do things that were out of my comfort zone. Unfortunately, that also meant having to experience extreme episodes of anxiety before, sometimes during, and definitely after a particular event or initiative. I was interviewed on radio shows, gave university lectures, ran corporate foot clinics, performed golf fitness assessments and spent weekends at health expos offering posture screenings.

On the surface, I had so many things to be grateful for – wife, kids, friends, career, travel, sports, music, and on and on. It is almost easy to see why I was so frustrated. How could I not be grateful for all of that?

In reality, though, I was grateful. I was also incoherent in so many ways and it was affecting my ability to self-regulate, reduce my stress level and alleviate the anxiety I was experiencing. I literally couldn't feel the gratitude I knew was there.

Over time, I lost the ability to feel anything other than anxiety. I didn't feel emotions anymore. I didn't get angry at someone. I got anxious. I didn't feel the emotions of sadness or guilt. I felt anxious. Every emotion I felt was expressed as anxiety. I felt incoherent with so many aspects of my life such as my relationships, my diet and my sense of self. Some people experienced anger, deep depression or became alcoholics. I got anxious. The incoherence in my life was manifesting as anxiety.

I felt like I was living a double life. In some areas, I was extremely confident and would seek out and embrace leadership roles. I had confidence in my ability and competence as a chiropractor. I was confident when I played sports. I felt calm and in charge when speaking in front of audiences or one-on-one with a patient. When I felt comfortable enough to be myself, I exuded confidence. I felt like a leader.

The juxtaposition of being a passionate speaker and doctor versus the person coping with, at times, debilitating symptoms was my energy-draining reality. Anxiety is what defined me for many years. Sometimes it was unrelenting for weeks or months at a time. It affected all aspects of my life.

Over the years, some friends distanced themselves from me and at times, I distanced myself from others. It was hurtful when I didn't feel supported. It took a long time to release the resentment I felt. Thankfully, as I healed, I was able to see a bigger picture. Everyone did the best they could. Some people had their own health issues or challenges with their family, some people had difficulty seeing me suffer and some people just made the best choices they could for themselves at the time.

In my thirties, while building my practice at York University and then in Midtown Toronto, it was challenging to live a double life. I felt passionate and uplifted when I was with my patients but as soon as I had a break, I'd shut my door and pretty much fall apart. I even cried some mornings on my way in. I didn't want to be there and I spent most of the day focused on when I could go home. The irony was that the only time I was actually in the moment and the only time I didn't feel debilitating anxiety was when I was with a patient and focused on our interaction. So that is what I did.

I have never missed a day of work due to anxiety. It may have been torturous at times but I had several things going for me. I knew, inherently, that being there and engaging with people was the best thing for me. It took a lot of emotional energy to get there but I felt like myself when I was engaged with patients.

The other motivating factor was my fear of losing everything if I didn't keep going. I dreaded financial ruin, losing friends and family, and the thought that I just couldn't keep up.

Fortunately for me, as I was helping people heal, I was helping myself at the same time. It was such a gift to be able to use the mindfulness and focus of helping someone else, to reduce my suffering and provide me the opportunity to engage in life.

Being a Chiropractor

In some ways, being a chiropractor has been a perfect fit for me. Chiropractors, by nature, are always looking for ways to improve, excel, be accepted, legitimized, respected and understood. Sounds like me, right?

Chiropractic care is powerful! Thankfully, scientific research is finally in catch-up mode and is uncovering the neurological and energetic impact of an adjustment. I thrive on seeing people's health transform and I'm grateful to be a part of their changing paradigm.

Chiropractic care provides millions of people every day with an opportunity to reach their optimal health potential and live a happy, pain-free life. I am a passionate believer in the benefits of chiropractic care. I am simultaneously aware of the insecurities that come with the profession.

The existing medical establishment has made it very difficult for chiropractors to gain true, widespread acceptance. Confusion often arises as a result of ignorance and misinformation. I have spent endless hours finding the best methods to educate the community about the true benefits of chiropractic care.

There are certainly many successful and inspiring chiropractors who have risen to the top of the profession. They have overcome the obstacles chiropractors face by having a massive amount of confidence, intention and drive. They keep laser focused on their purpose to fuel their success.

The sad truth is that there are many skilled chiropractors, brilliant doctors, struggling to build their practice, when they should have lines around the corner.

When I became a chiropractor, I could have been anything I wanted. I was an exceptional student who earned great marks. Despite the anxiety I experienced, I was driven to succeed and I had a lot of confidence in my ability to do so. I wanted to choose a profession that I could enjoy on a daily basis and one that gave me the opportunity to explore my passions.

I had other professions on my list such as physiotherapy, architecture and law. I remember specifically not wanting to go into medicine. Funny enough, it wasn't because I had a problem with medication. It was far more simplistic. I just didn't want to spend the majority of my day looking in people's throats and listening to them tell me about their bowel movements.

Other than seeing a chiropractor to help with some back pain, I didn't know a lot about the background of chiropractic before I applied. I knew it was a profession that involved keeping the spine healthy and caring for people with musculoskeletal injuries. I was unaware there were different factions of chiropractors and that some had aligned themselves with the medical profession to try and gain acceptance.

As I became more educated, I learned that there was an entirely different aspect of chiropractic care that focused on the philosophy and intention behind the chiropractic adjustment. It was ironic, really, that when I made my decision, I had no idea there was a spiritual or philosophical aspect to chiropractic care that would end up being so inspiring to me.

The original goal of a chiropractic adjustment was to remove interference in the nervous system that was impeding the body's ability to heal and self-regulate. Healing, as we were taught in Chiropractic College, came from above down and from the inside out.

As I was beginning my chiropractic journey, I was also in the middle of transitioning from my life as a teen hippie into a respectable young adult. Choosing chiropractic as a profession resonated with me as I could continue my philosophical journey and maintain the principles I had learned regarding peace, love and good vibrations.

There was also the practical and physical aspect to the profession. Performing a chiropractic adjustment is similar to martial arts. There are technical aspects I enjoy practicing, that take time to master. There is always more to learn because there are a wide variety of techniques that address every aspect of the spine and nervous system. I've always been motivated to continue my learning and become an expert in as many techniques as possible.

In my career as a chiropractor, there have been several things I was unprepared for. Most people that initiate care in my office are either misinformed or uninformed about what chiropractors do and how we can help. That's a problem. In my experience, other doctors and therapists are also confused as to what chiropractors do and are hesitant to refer people for treatment.

In many cases, it is necessary to dispel and clarify the information my patients have been given by other practitioners. In these instances, it is important to explain why the information they received about chiropractic care is wrong. It can be quite challenging to educate someone while contradicting another health practitioner they already trust.

For most chiropractors, success depends on one's ability to communicate effectively. Working with many coaches and participating in business development programs helped me develop these skills.

As I look back at my journey, it is clear that I used my thirties and early forties to learn techniques and concepts that would eventually define the direction of my life as well as my career. It became harder and harder to distinguish whether I was learning and educating myself for personal or professional purposes. It didn't matter though because I was passionate about both.

Section 2

EXPLORATION AND DISCOVERY

In this section, I will discuss and delve into some of the most impactful concepts and healing techniques I've discovered and that have been instrumental in my life.

For the most part, people develop their life paradigm and the lens through which they view the world both from their parents and the environment in which they grew up. Many people begin to question their beliefs as they grow older, especially if they struggle in specific areas such as their career, relationships, chronic illness, stress or the general uncertainty of life.

As we created the *Coherence Revolution*, we knew there were many people who have some experience with breathwork, self-regulation techniques and stress relief strategies. Some people will have come across these concepts, know the language and read many books on the subject of healing. This program is definitely for those people. If you are one of them, I encourage you to explore all the suggested links and resources so you get the most out of the program.

We also created the program for people who are new to these concepts. We wanted to be an access point into the world of self-actualization, personal growth, quantum healing and the world of *coherence* for those intrigued by the topics and who seek a true understanding of the power of these concepts.

We designed this course to save you thousands of dollars and endless hours of searching. Our hope is that you can start to add coherence into your life immediately, no matter where you are on your journey.

My intention for discussing all of these impactful concepts, therapies, books and courses is to share my experiences and offer insight and inspiration through my challenges and successes.

My hope is that your new understanding will have a powerful and lasting effect on how you perceive the world around you and how you choose to interact with it.

Chapter 9

WHAT IS HEALTH?

I would have to say that the predominant focus of my adult life has been the pursuit of *getting healthy*. Due to my choice of career and my personal journey, the meaning of *getting healthy* has been redefined many times. For most people, it's a source of confusion. Does it mean you should focus on each individual health concern? Do you need treatment or therapy to achieve health? What is the best approach to eliminate physical symptoms, ailments, disease, anxiety, stress or depression?

What is health? Perhaps it's easier to start with what it's not.

Health is definitely not just the absence of symptoms. Unfortunately, most people do base their health on how they look and how they feel. If they feel good and look good, then the assumption is that they must be healthy. If they feel pain or symptoms, then the assumption is that they are not well.

Nothing could be further from the truth.

Health is more accurately defined in terms of *optimal function*. When every cell, tissue and organ in the body is functioning, healing and replicating perfectly, you are in a state of health. Health is the process of functioning optimally.

Take heart disease for example. What is the first symptom of heart disease? In 80% of the cases, the first symptom of heart disease is death due to a heart attack. By the time you realize there is a problem, it's already too late!

In general, when dealing with chronic health concerns, the symptoms are the last things to appear. The disease process actually begins a long time before any of the symptoms manifest.

When a stressor overwhelms the nervous system's ability to adapt optimally, a process of dis-ease begins. As these stressors accumulate and the systems continue to function improperly, the state of dis-ease causes more widespread dysfunction throughout the body.

When there is repetitive and sustained dysfunction of the cells and tissues, over time it reduces the body's repair and replication capabilities. In other words, your cells are not healing or reproducing properly. When that occurs, the process is now called *disease*.

Here's another common example to illustrate that *being healthy* refers to the process of optimal function.

Let's say you eat a chicken sandwich for lunch and within a few hours begin to feel ill and start vomiting. Over the next 24 hours, you experience all the symptoms you would expect in this scenario, including a fever and diarrhea. Would you say you were sick or healthy?

If you haven't guessed it, you had food poisoning. If you were truly sick, what would have happened? You would have died! What you ate was poison. And you didn't die because your body was operating as it should have, and the poison was recognized and then removed. Your body was healthy enough to rid itself of the toxin.

When defining *health*, I think it's crucial to discuss it in terms of a process and a dynamic *state of being* rather than an end goal you are trying to achieve. You are a healthy person when every cell, tissue and organ in your body function optimally. That is when each system is harmonious and aligned with every other system in your body.

The human body is exposed and adapts to a variety of stressors every day. Whether the stressor is your diet, medication, desk posture, sport injury or relationship issue, the more effectively you adapt, the less impact it will have on your health.

You are healthy when your body is able to adapt efficiently, process information effectively and create a response that results in optimal function.

Your ability to adapt to stress will determine the level of health you can maintain. All types of stress are cumulative and the human body can only tolerate so much stress (what's called the allostatic load: see Appendix) before the nervous system overloads. Similar to a computer, we have to shut down and reboot or we risk causing more serious, long-term damage.

According to research done in the field of epigenetics (see Appendix), stress literally affects your genes. Whether you have gone through a divorce, were fired from your job, had a car accident, ate too much processed food, lived beside an electrical power plant, smoked cigarettes or sat at your desk all day, that stress can and will overload your nervous system and ultimately lead to sickness and disease.

So I'd like you to clarify even further, what does health mean to you? Is your goal to be symptom free? Do you want to feel healthy? Are you trying to improve your function? Is your intention to increase your level of coherence?

Obviously, being healthy is a core goal for most people, but how long can your body stay healthy and function optimally if you are incoherent?

Health and happiness are much easier to achieve and perhaps more importantly, to sustain, when you become familiar with all of the large and small momentary choices you can make to facilitate health. If you spend your time with people or engage in activities that help evoke the feeling of being *in the zone*, or feeling more like your authentic self, it results in a renewing emotional response. It's that positive emotional response that facilitates healthier functioning in the body. When it comes to health, it's not the destination – it's the process. The more often your body is in a state of health, the better you will feel and the more effectively you will heal.

Chapter 10

IMPACTFUL DISCOVERIES

PSYCH-K®

Created and developed by Dr. Bruce Lipton and Rob Williams, PSYCH-K is a revolutionary technique that helps you discover and replace self-limiting subconscious belief patterns.

I first discovered this method of healing while reading Dr. Lipton's book, *The Biology of Belief*. It is one of the first books I recommend to anyone wanting a good foundation and understanding of the quantum view of health. I was intrigued by his perspective and his pioneering work in the field of *epigenetics* (see Appendix). I inherently knew that my thoughts and beliefs were affecting my behavior.

The concepts in this book helped me understand the power and impact of repetitive negative thought patterns on our subconscious mind. For example, if you habitually tell yourself you are *not good enough,* it can become a virtually unbreakable neurological connection. With repetition, a powerful subconscious belief program will be installed that will run in the background of everything you do, always.

The technique PSYCH-K brought all of these concepts to life. It provided practical meaning and made me keenly aware of how much damage was caused from the repetitive thoughts and insecurities I developed growing up. I always knew that the messages I was giving myself did not serve me well and learning how to use PSYCH-K allowed me to explore that aspect of myself.

The technique helps you discover and understand your subconscious beliefs, which gives you the opportunity to choose which ones to keep or replace. It's up to you. You choose. During a PSYCH-K session, a form of muscle testing is used as a means of communication with the body.

There are many ways to muscle test and many explanations of what to do and why it works. In general, when your subconscious beliefs don't match your conscious beliefs, your ability to create a strong muscle contraction weakens. When you are holding an item that depletes you, thinking a thought or uttering words that are in the negative, your muscle firing will weaken.

Muscle testing can be used for many reasons, but as it pertains to PSYCH-K, the first step is to ask your subconscious questions and determine your belief systems based on the strength of your arm's resistance. The second aspect of PSYCH-K is a technique that facilitates uploading new, healthy belief systems or perceptions.

In our family, we frequently use muscle testing to help us understand our thoughts, habits and food sensitivities. In much the same way as subconscious beliefs can cause a weakened muscle contraction, so can foods, places or objects. If a food is not coherent with your body on a cellular level, your body will respond with weakened muscle firing.

From a coherence perspective, it's important to know what is incoherent. Muscle testing can be a great asset especially if you're looking to do an elimination diet. Periodically I will experience a lot of anxiety after a meal, and by using muscle testing, I am able to understand which foods or chemicals are incoherent with my body. Then, if necessary, I am able to do an elimination diet to confirm if the food should be avoided.

Over the years I've had a lot of success using PSYCH-K with patients to help them reprogram their subconscious belief patterns in many different areas. I have seen people, who were on the verge of giving up, heal quicker, overcome themselves and accomplish goals that didn't seem possible.

It simply isn't possible to be in coherence when your subconscious is running automatic programs based on negative belief systems. PSYCH-K makes it possible to create new and healthy subconscious belief systems.

I've used PSYCH-K with hundreds of people over the last 15 years. Everyone has had their own motivation for seeking me out, but ultimately, the majority of people have the same negative subconscious belief patterns that deal with self-acceptance and self-love.

Muscle testing example 1

Patient: 12-year-old boy

Concern: stress, anxiety, difficulty adapting, defiance when he doesn't feel safe

Situation: He didn't feel the need to participate in art class and expressed his frustration with having to participate in something he saw no need for.

I believed that he was nervous to fail and had no confidence in his creative abilities but wanted to know why. As I began muscle testing, I quickly received some feedback that led me to start asking his subconscious questions about his past education and teachers. The reason I am including this example in the book is because it was one of the biggest a-ha moments you could have when working with someone.

Outcomes

STRONG response: When the muscle contraction is strong, that suggests the conscious and subconscious mind are in agreement.

WEAK response: When the muscle contraction is weak, that suggests there is a disagreement between the conscious and subconscious mind. Negative statements and beliefs will cause a weakened contraction as will anything that your subconscious believes is untrue.

Patient interaction

Muscle Test: 'I am good at art.'

WEAK: He could not hold his arm up.

Muscle Test: 'Someone told me I was bad at art.'

STRONG: He could easily resist my attempt to push his arm down.

Muscle Test: 'My parents told me I was bad at art.'

WEAK.

Muscle Test: 'A teacher told me I was bad at art.'

STRONG.

Muscle Test: 'Grade 4' – WEAK. 'Grade 3' – WEAK. 'Grade 2' – STRONG. 'Kindergarten' – WEAK.

Muscle Test: 'My grade 2 teacher told me I was bad at art.'

STRONG.

Eureka! I will paraphrase his reaction. And yes, it was practically one big, long sentence that just came flying out.

'Oh yeah, my second grade teacher, Ms. S. [not real] told me I wasn't good enough and that I couldn't draw because I needed more time to finish my piece of art, and the girl beside me finished two days ago and the teacher compared me to her and said mine wasn't good enough. I have been embarrassed ever since.' He looked at me and gave me a high five. It was brilliant.

We hadn't even done any actual corrections or uploaded any new beliefs. Simply facilitating the understanding elicited a strong emotional response that resulted in a change in behavior. He agreed to participate and give his best effort in class.

Over several months, we worked together, using PSYCH-K, to create subconscious belief patterns that supported and encouraged confidence and healthy self-esteem.

Muscle testing example 2

Patient: 35-year-old woman

Scenario: As a chiropractor, I use muscle testing as an additional objective measure to determine if my patient's nervous system is balanced. Sometimes I feel like there are more areas of the spine to address and I find it useful to assess the situation through a different lens.

In this example, the woman presented with lower back pain and it hurt to lift her legs while lying down on her stomach. After I adjusted her, she was still unable to lift her right leg, mostly due to a feeling of heaviness and lack of control over the movement. In situations such as this, muscle testing helps guide me to the solution.

Muscle Test: 'My body is completely balanced for today.'

WEAK.

Muscle Test: 'Another adjustment would be optimal.'

STRONG.

Cervical: WEAK.

Thoracic: STRONG.

Lumbar: WEAK.

T1–6 (meaning the first through sixth thoracic vertebra): WEAK.

T7–12: STRONG.

T7 (WEAK), T8 (WEAK), T9 (WEAK), T10 (WEAK), T11 (WEAK), T12 (STRONG).

Adjust while lying on back: WEAK.

Adjust while lying on stomach: STRONG.

I had her lie on her stomach. I adjusted her T12 vertebra very gently, and almost as soon as my hand recoiled from the adjustment, her leg flew up. Her power was restored and the pain was gone. I have learned to listen to the body because of powerful moments such as this.

———————————

Reconnective Healing®

In April of 2005, I participated in a workshop given by Dr. Eric Pearle, an author, chiropractor and energy healer who trained health practitioners in Reconnective Healing®. It was a memorable few days for many reasons, not least of which was that it coincided with the first week of my daughter Jessica's life.

In my mind, there was a dual purpose for attending the workshop, which happened to be a common theme for every therapy, self-help, growth and inspirational experience I've had. I was both desperate to heal and fascinated by the approach to healing. Every time I discovered a new healing modality, I wanted to explore how it could be used to improve my own health and at the same time, help me become a better chiropractor.

I was always searching and wondering if the next option would finally be the cure. Would it be the solution that eliminated the anxiety I experienced? Will it give me the opportunity to live a normal life?

Once I read about a new concept or attended a seminar involving a new technique or therapy, I became curious and I wanted to experience it. I definitely had an open mind and tended to want to trust the information I read. I think being critical is very important, but I have also found that being too critical can be limiting. As long as I researched and determined that the approach I was exploring was safe, I tried it. If it helped, at that point, I would delve deeper to learn more and find out why it was helping me.

I deeply cared about *the why*. My scientific and rational mind desperately wanted to understand how and why something was going to help me. Unfortunately, at times I felt the urgent need for quick relief. In those cases, as long as I knew I wouldn't do any damage by trying it, the research and understanding came later.

Dr. Pearle's workshop was no different. I met Dr. Pearle in Las Vegas at a chiropractic seminar a year prior to the workshop he offered in Toronto. I attended one of his lectures and witnessed how he completely blew everyone away with his manipulation of energy and the healings he facilitated with people in the audience.

One evening, he saw my friends and I at a blackjack table and approached us. He started to joke around a bit and seemed to feel a connection between us. We shared a common culture and educational background so there was a natural comfort level.

When I found out he was coming to Toronto, I knew I had to go.

It was a paradigm-shifting three days that was spent learning about and playing with energy. Initially, I had a hard time buying into some of the activities he had us engage in such as partnering up with someone to practice throwing and catching energy. We used our imagination to envision throwing a ball of energy back and forth. I felt very silly doing it at first, but as the weekend progressed and I had the opportunity to witness him facilitate the movement of energy through people's bodies, I was convinced. I may not have known exactly what was happening, but I knew I was learning something very powerful. I witnessed people tremble and shake from the tips of their toes to the top of their head.

Many people who were the recipients of energy work shared their experiences of seeing swirling colours and incredible visions. Hearing these perspectives and experiences fascinated me.

On the last day of the workshop, we were divided into pairs and practiced energy work on one another. We took turns using our hands to sense different frequencies around our partner's body. The intention was to simply play with and observe the energy.

As a technical side note, it's important to understand that during a session of Reconnective Healing®, the practitioner monitors the strength of the sensation they feel in the palm of their own hands. One of the unique aspects of Reconnective Healing® is that the feeling in the practitioner's palms can increase as they move further away from the patient. When this occurs, the patient also has a more profound experience.

Considering my more recent experiences with meditation and energy work, the experience with Dr. Pearle actually makes more sense to me now than it did then. The intention of playing with energetic frequencies wasn't to create a healing. It was to help facilitate increased coherence within our partners as well as ourselves.

I worked on my partner for a few minutes with limited expectations, but to my surprise, my partner began to shake. It wasn't just a normal shake. Both his eyes were twitching at different rhythms and his body started to gyrate aggressively.

I continued to focus on the sensation I was feeling in the middle of my palms as I moved further away from his body. Imagine having a piece of gum stuck to your palm as you start to pull on it. The more you pull on the gum, the stronger the gum pulls on your skin. That's what the frequencies felt like. The further I moved my hands away from my partner, the more intense the sensation was in my hands.

Initially, it startled and surprised me, so instinctively, I dropped my hands. His body instantly became still. People around the room began to gather around my table and Dr. Pearle stood by my side to see what I would do next.

I took a deep breath, used my hands to reconnect with the energy and pulled back. Just like the first time, he started to vibrate and twitch on the table. I played for a few more minutes and then put my hands down to let my partner rest and recover.

That was the first time I witnessed someone processing coherent energy.

Feng shui

I was first interested in feng shui around 2007. I was intrigued and wanted to understand as much as I could about the flow of energy. I did some research on the subject to help me decide the best way to proceed. Eventually I decided to dive right in, so I bought a home course called Diamond Feng Shui. The course focused on how to assess your living space and develop methods to increase good energy flow in all aspects of your life.

At first, I was pretty committed. I read each chapter intently and completed the homework. I made quite a few changes to my space, wrote affirmations on what I envisioned for my life and placed them all over my home and work environments.

I was dedicated for a while. However, it only lasted a few months. Some of the learning became very time consuming. I wasn't seeing any quick changes that I could attribute to feng shui. Eventually it became just another initiative that didn't last very long. However, like so many things in my life, it made a comeback!

As an antidote to feeling stuck, I revisited feng shui in the summer of 2015. I had so many good things in my life, truly a framework for success, yet I was still struggling with anxiety and unable to achieve the success in my career that I expected. I seemed to be doing all the right things but still not getting the results I was looking for.

I brought the original feng shui course back out to see if I could try again and hopefully achieve better results. I started the program pretty much where I left off and quickly got frustrated again because the changes weren't happening quick enough.

I determined that if I was going to achieve results with feng shui, I was going to have to hire an expert. My wife Aviva and I consulted with a few feng shui practitioners and eventually hired someone to come give us advice on how to apply feng shui to both our house and my business.

The practitioner made some suggestions for every room and area of our home. We put a comprehensive plan together and tried to follow each of her suggestions. Some of the changes resonated with us while some felt very forced. I knew I was engaging in the process out of desperation rather than a sense of enthusiasm and playfulness.

Even though we had mixed feelings about our experience, the concept of feng shui made a lot of sense to me. It still does. It's another way to talk about coherence and facilitating the flow of energy.

I'm very happy that I've dabbled in the art of feng shui and can utilize the concepts to reinforce the power and impact of coherent energy. It has taught me to be mindful and aware of how I can optimize the flow of energy in my surroundings.

These are a few takeaways from the course that I still use to this day.

Always face the door while sitting at your desk. You should always be able to see who and what comes through the door. If you are like me, it doesn't feel right to have your back facing the door.

Use mirrors in hallways or reflective images to make sure the energy keeps moving through the home and doesn't stagnate anywhere.

Always arrange your bed so that it is facing the door. Similar to a desk, you should always be able to see someone coming in.

BrainTap®

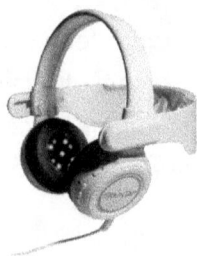

As I spent time studying and training in brain-based healing techniques, I was exposed to a wide range of neurologically based healing modalities. I also had the opportunity to explore and try unique and revolutionary products.

Of all the products, there was one that resonated with me the most. BrainTap is a form of neurofeedback that ultimately helps reduce and neutralize stress on the brain. The technology combines the use of light, sound, binaural beats, laser technology and guided meditation. There are hundreds of different sessions which are usually each just under a half hour. Some of the more popular topics included are chronic pain, sleep issues, stress, anxiety, weight loss, coping with cancer, alcoholism, healthy children, strengthened immune system and many more. Over time and with consistent use, it helps facilitate more coherent brain patterns. A 20-minute session actually provides the brain with the equivalent rest of a 3.5-hour nap. Even after one session, the brain has a chance to reset.

I began using BrainTap with patients before or after their regular adjustments. Due to the wide range of topics that are offered through the sessions, it gave me an opportunity to change the type of conversation I was having with them. People began to tell me how they felt about many aspects of their lives. I started to hear about the stress people felt in their lives and it seemed to give people permission to discuss other health issues such as chronic headaches, eating and sleep disorders, addictions, mental health issues, heart disease and even cancer.

People understand the concept of *stress causing disease* and are generally open to anything that will help them reduce it. My patients were excited to learn about the benefits and open to trying the technology. The results have consistently been incredible. I love hearing about their initial experience. The most common response I receive is that they were finally able to relax. Some people fall asleep. Some people think it's only been five minutes and others take a few minutes to process being awake, similar to waking up from a good nap.

Each BrainTap session helps create new, positive subconscious belief changes that become hardwired with repetition. It transports my patients out of their typical day and provides them with a unique experience. Sometimes that's enough to make it valuable. BrainTap is much more though. I have consistently received incredible feedback from patients who improved their sleep, reduced anxiety, changed their mood, lost weight, eliminated their headaches and that's just to name a few. I've been able to help people in ways I was never able to before.

Dr. Joe Dispenza

In mid-2016, a friend told me about a seminar he attended that taught meditation and concepts that focused on energy and quantum physics. He also added that it was so much more. I was intrigued.

He mentioned the name of the doctor who ran the seminar. It sounded familiar. It turned out that I had seen a couple movies he had been in. His name was Dr. Joe Dispenza.

I did a bit of research on Dr. Joe, and I was fascinated by his journey and the work he was doing. I ended up going out to buy two books, *Breaking the Habit of Being Yourself* and *You Are the Placebo*. When I went to put them away, what did I see? One of his earlier books, *Evolve Your Brain,* was sitting in my personal library. I knew it all sounded so familiar.

Over the next several months, I read the books and practiced the meditations daily. I was hooked. By the end of the summer my wife, Aviva, and I booked our first three-day workshop for December of 2016 in Philadelphia. We committed to practicing the work daily, which actually took a significant amount of willpower. We weren't just sitting down to do a quick ten-minute meditation. The meditations we started with were slightly over an hour.

The three-day workshop was life changing. It was the fuel and inspiration that motivated us to continue the journey at home and at future events. With each subsequent event, the intensity built for us. We followed up the three-day with a five-day event the following year. In 2018 and 2019, we took it to the next level and attended a couple of seven-day retreats.

The workshops have been a microcosm of my life. Over the course of just a few days, my emotional landscape fluctuated from depleting to renewing energies and from lack of self-esteem to confidence. I've had some extreme highs but also some really raw and personal lows. Each workshop has been precisely planned with plenty of opportunities to face your demons and overcome yourself.

At some of the workshops, when I joined groups of people, it felt like my high school experience all over again. There was the perceived 'cool group,' the 'weird' people and the 'misfits.' At different events and in different situations, I experienced feeling like each of them. Back and forth it went, and I was consciously aware of it the whole time. I watched and listened to myself make decisions for the day as I entered the workshop. I decided where to sit based on my assumptions of people. I helped people who looked confused and made people feel comfortable. I cracked a joke and explained a concept to the group. I felt like the healer and then like the one who needed healing. My sense of self always fluctuated based on my external environment.

With experience came awareness. The more aware I was that this was going on, the more I started to control my responses.

Once I understood I was just replaying old neural patterns, I started to break them down. I began transforming my emotional response consciously, which helped me achieve a more coherent state. As my emotional state elevated and I felt more renewing emotions, my perception of the events going on around me shifted.

It became much less about trying to control the environment and those around me, and more about controlling my inner environment in healthy, conscious and awakened states.

Once that happened, and I was consciously practicing other ways to react, I would literally look around at the crowd through different eyes. I was starting to get better at using the new tools and techniques I was learning to improve my own experience at the seminar.

I have come to understand that the process of solving a problem does not actually start by trying to solve the problem. That is not the first step. First, we must become more coherent and then we can reassess the situation, being able to see it through new eyes – coherent eyes.

Since starting Dr. Joe's work in 2016, one of my goals has been to create a habit of opening my heart and listening to others. The more I've done that, the more I've realized that most people are just doing their best to get through their life. I now recognize that it was my incoherent belief systems that caused me to cast judgments on others.

I've often been hard on myself for being judgmental of others. How could I judge someone else when I was experiencing my own inner turmoil? In reality, if you analyze the types of things you're judgmental about, you realize that most of the time, those judgments are the mind's attempt to protect you from perceived danger in the form of rejection and embarrassment.

Many of the insecure assumptions I made repeatedly over the years were based on past stories I told myself that may not even have relevance anymore. When I began to consciously listen to what people were telling me, it was obvious that many of the stories I told myself did not resemble the truth or reflect the intentions from the other person's perspective.

The more aware we become of our thoughts, the less likely we are to continue running our old programs. One of the many benefits I've received from attending Dr. Joe's weeklong events is that they gave me the opportunity to dismantle some of my hardwired programming which were created through the perception of a teenage boy. Take for instance the experiences I had trying to figure out who to sit beside. Every morning when we showed up and entered the hall to join our group, I scanned the area to figure out which seat to choose. Until I felt comfortable in a group, I was generally self-conscious in those types of situations. It was a leftover program that was over 30 years old. I wanted to identify the people who seemed to be liked by everyone. I was anxious to see who would choose to sit with me. I really wanted to know who would validate me. My thoughts would have me believe that if I could just figure out who those people were, then I'd have a great workshop and a powerful breakthrough. Obviously, that is not the way it works, but those are truly the thoughts that were going through my mind. My brain would do its best to bombard me with every possible fearful and insecure thought.

I'm sure you're not surprised to hear this, but I never accomplished my goal of finding the perfect person to sit beside using that method of thinking. I did, however, find the perfect person every single time. In retrospect, that became very clear. I learned a lot of important lessons from each of the people I sat beside or spent time with at all of the events.

Dr. Joe's work has been instrumental in my growth and continues to inspire me. Of all the habits and modalities I've engaged in over the years, this is perhaps the first practice I went all-in. I haven't questioned why I want to do it or if I should do it at any point. It has always felt *coherent*.

Soma breathwork

During Christmas break in 2019, I was scanning through my Facebook feed when I came across an ad for a breathwork course called *Soma*. After watching a few videos and reading the educational materials, I decided to purchase the course with Aviva.

The concepts taught as part of the Soma technique are extremely congruent with the breathwork taught by HeartMath, Dr. Joe Dispenza and as I found out later, Wim Hof. I became more and more fascinated by all of the different breathwork techniques. The idea of being able to regulate the parasympathetic nervous system by using different frequencies and intensities of breathing and breath retention resonated with me. It made perfect sense that, as humans, we could access our self-regulating and self-healing capabilities through the most accessible tool we have – our breath.

Aviva and I completed the course together and found it pretty easy to learn and practice. I enjoyed all the tingly sensations I felt during and after a session. I also liked the fact that there was research backing up the science behind the technique. I often practiced while using a pulse oximeter to monitor my oxygen saturation levels. I found it very powerful to be able to track and measure my progress. Soma was instrumental in my process of learning and understanding how much control we have over our own nervous system.

Wim Hof breathwork

Sometimes in life, things seemingly happen due to chance. While in other circumstances, the timing feels like it was divinely planned. Although I had watched a few videos about Wim Hof and knew of his technique, I was properly introduced to the Wim Hof Method shortly after taking the Soma course.

I had heard of Wim Hof and knew a bit of his story, but I had never looked into doing his program. Then the COVID-19 pandemic hit. Literally the day after I had to close down my clinic, I saw an advertisement on Facebook for the Wim Hof Method and it was 50% off! That was enough to motivate me to take action. The description of the ten-week course seemed pretty intense, and both Aviva and I were excited to dive in.

I found Wim Hof, the creator of the method, to have a unique blend of knowledge, humor, intrigue, possibility, science and silliness. What feels the most satisfying to me about the Wim Hof Method is that it is simple, and it is effective.

There are two key aspects to the Wim Hof Method that have proved to be extremely powerful for me as tools to break the feeling of anxiety and neutralize stress. The Wim Hof Method encompasses specific breathwork techniques as well as the use of cold to help the body self-regulate the parasympathetic nervous system.

The course includes training for both cold showers and ice baths. While my initial experiences with cold showers were a bit shocking to my system, they are now a welcome awakening to my body, mind and spirit.

The Wim Hof Method is definitely one of the most impactful habits and routines I have implemented as part of my personal Coherence Revolution.

Zero Limits / Ho'oponopono

Ho'oponopono focuses on repentance, forgiveness, gratitude and love.

Practice Ho'oponopono by saying:
'I'm sorry. Please forgive me. Thank you. I love you.'

Joe Vitale's book is a thorough and well-thought-out introduction to Ho'oponopono. I have always found it amusing and fascinating while also admiring the simplicity and sophistication of the healing technique.

Ho'oponopono is a very simple yet tedious technique. It's repetitive. The main process consists of repeating four important phrases: 'I love you,' 'Thank you,' 'Forgive me,' 'I'm sorry.' The process of saying these four phrases over and over again is called *cleaning*. Repeating the phrases *cleans* the subconscious beliefs and circumstances in your life that are holding you back from living the life you've dreamed of. *Cleaning* means that you essentially revert to your pure source or consciousness, which is in the present moment. It's an interesting concept because you can and you are encouraged to clean for anything that shows up in your consciousness even if it's someone else's problem. If you are aware of it, then you can *clean* on it.

The objective of Ho'oponopono is to *clean* unwanted thoughts and beliefs from your conscious and subconscious mind and ultimately, from existence.

It is human nature to notice things in others you would like to change or to have situations that you would like to avoid. Ho'oponopono can certainly be used to create external change, but your intention should not be to *clean* others. The goal is always to *clean* your own consciousness. Taking responsibility for anything that shows up in your consciousness provides you the opportunity to *clean* it. Imagine if everyone took personal responsibility for an issue like global warming, as if each of our actions and behaviors were part of the problem. Each of us can be part of the solution by practicing Ho'oponopono. What a different world it could be.

As I've practiced Ho'oponopono, I've tried to understand why those four particular phrases were chosen: thank you, I love you, forgive me, I am sorry.

What I realized is that it isn't so much about understanding why, as much as it is about being able to connect them to my life in an authentic way.

Practicing Ho'oponopono regularly helps create a habit of focusing on your heart and also reminds you of the importance of word choice even when speaking to yourself. Whether you say the words in your head or out loud, they have a huge impact on both you and the individual they are directed at.

The reason this technique resonates with me is because I see immense value in the core principle, which is to take 100% responsibility for everything in your life. I also like that as you engage in the technique, the positive words you repeat facilitate an immediate change in your mindset. That alone can be enough of a neurological interrupt to change the negative or stressful situation which requires cleaning.

When your goal is to clean all the negative beliefs, habits and patterns you have developed, then every opportunity to clean is welcome. Every time anxiety is triggered, or you experience a stressful, unwanted situation, it can be seen as an opportunity to clean. Every time you see something in someone else that frustrates you, it's an opportunity to clean. Once you are able to see your challenges as opportunities, the intensity of the trigger is automatically reduced.

Ho'oponopono has helped me learn how to feel gratitude even in difficult situations. When issues or triggers arise, I'm grateful to have the opportunity to clean because that means the issue is on its way out.

During the COVID-19 pandemic, as I was writing and developing this course, I decided to get certified in Ho'oponopono. I had read the book *Zero Limits* and practiced Ho'oponopono on and off for several years, and it felt like the right time to dive deeper. Intuitively, I felt like the technique resonated with my goals and intention to learn how to open my heart.

Getting certified required me to watch hours of video from a Ho'oponopono workshop. Throughout the series of videos, the attendees asked questions about how to use the technique and how to respond to questions about the technique. The teacher, Dr. Hew Len, always responded the same way; he told them to *clean*. Thank you. Forgive me. I love you. I'm sorry.

No matter what the question was, that was his response.

It was intriguing. You could tell he had complete certainty in what he was teaching, and because of that, it was much easier for me to believe the information and the story he told.

In my opinion, Ho'oponopono can be a primary transformative tool. Simply saying the four phrases can elicit an emotional response. The words themselves resonate at a frequency that literally creates a positive physiologic change as you say them.

We know from the work of Masaru Emoto (*Hidden Messages in Water*) that words produce dramatically different cellular responses based upon whether their tone and connotation are energetically positive or energetically negative.

Integrating Ho'oponopono

Whether I am meditating, practicing HeartMath or simply being mindful, my goal is to consistently have a coherent, open heart.

For the heart to achieve a smooth coherent rhythm, several things are necessary: positive mental focus, a specific rhythmic breathing pattern and an ability to cultivate a renewing emotional state.

When I was completing the Ho'oponopono certification, I realized that when I practiced Ho'oponopono while using the HeartMath technology, I achieved greater coherence with less effort. I felt more open and able to connect to a positive emotion. I also had an overall sense that I was diving deeper into my daily meditations.

It was motivating and reassuring to know that by using the HeartMath technology, I was actually able to confirm that when I used Ho'oponopono, my heart and brain were, in fact, functioning in a more coherent state.

Section 3

COHERENCE

This section explores practical applications of coherence which build on the fundamental concepts developed by the HeartMath Institute and the work of Dr. Joe Dispenza, who have been pioneers in this field.

To get the most out of this section, I recommend you create a user profile at **www.coherencerevolution.com** where you will have access to videos and worksheets that will provide support along the way. Review the material as many times as you would like. There is no rush. Take your time and be mindful.

The *Coherence Revolution* live course provides an excellent opportunity to practice and refine all of the new habits, behaviors and skills you've learned. You can complete the *Coherence Revolution* live course at any point of your journey. It can be the push you need to make a change, or it can be a powerful experience after you have begun to embody the concepts you are learning. While the live experience is a separate and distinct program from the book, it is the summation of the key concepts of the *Coherence Revolution*. It is a natural progression from the book as it delves deeper and guides you through a journey of self-discovery, teaching you how to maximize coherence in every aspect of your life.

Chapter 11

HEARTMATH

The HeartMath® Institute was founded in 1991 as a non-profit research center to study the relationship between stress, emotion, brain, and heart function. They have done robust scientific research into the role of the heart in brain and nervous system function, stress and performance, and overall well-being.

As a result of their research, HeartMath has developed a range of practical techniques that can be used *in the moment* to prevent, neutralize, and recover from stress. They have also developed award-winning biofeedback and mobile stress reduction technology that can be used on your smartphone, tablet, or PC to *monitor* and *retrain* your heart rhythm patterns into a state of coherence.

According to the HeartMath Institute, *coherence* is 'an optimal state in which the heart, mind and emotions are operating in-sync and are balanced.'

HeartMath describes *coherence* as a state where physiologically, the immune, hormonal and nervous systems function in a state of energetic coordination.

Coherence is a scientific term that describes a highly efficient, health-promoting state associated with positive emotion and a high degree of mental and emotional stability. In other words, physiologically, there is heart alignment between your mental, emotional, spiritual and physical system and you feel balanced and energized.

Coherence is a scientific term for what psychologists call the *flow state* and athletes call being *in the zone*.

How can using HeartMath techniques help you?

The aim of using these techniques and technologies in one's daily health or spiritual practices is to increase psychophysiological coherence while lowering stress. This in turn enables greater creativity. 'The more you increase your coherence baseline, the more access you will have to your creative capacities,' according to HeartMath's research director, Rollin McCraty, PhD.

'HeartMath's positive emotion-focused techniques help individuals learn to self-generate and sustain a beneficial functional mode known as *psychophysiological coherence*, characterized by increased emotional stability and by increased synchronization and harmony in the functioning of physiological systems,' asserts Dr. McCraty.

Research conducted evaluating the efficacy of the HeartMath system for generating coherence has demonstrated the following:

- improved brain function,
- increased ability to self-regulate,
- improvement in long-term memory,
- improvement in short-term memory,
- increased ability to focus,
- increased ability to process information,

- increased reaction times,

- higher test scores,

- stronger immune system,

- easier recovery,

- increased capacity to build resilience and energy reserves.

———————————

My first official introduction to the concept of coherence was in 2005, through my introduction to HeartMath. It was a time of growth, and I was discovering so many new books and healing modalities around this time.

While browsing through the self-help section at Indigo, a book caught my eye. I was really attracted to the concept of regulating my emotions and eliminating my anxiety using my breath. I understood the concept on a very basic level but I didn't understand how profound the state of coherence could be. Something about the technique felt right. It was simple, natural, and it could be practiced anywhere at any time.

As was common in my journey, I could see how beneficial this technique would be for me and for my patients. I remember being intrigued enough that I ordered two versions of the biofeedback technology right from the start. One for home and one for the office. I practiced almost daily for quite a while.

At that point, my understanding of coherence was limited to breathing slower and deeper to help facilitate a state of calm. I understood on an intellectual level why coherence was important and that I experienced an uplifting feeling in my body when I had a smoother breathing rhythm. I had minimal experience at the time of how to use emotion to change my physiological state but I started experimenting with that concept and was doing my best to practice feeling different emotions. I felt like I was putting in a lot of effort and I had the right attitude.

At the time I thought I was improving. In hindsight, I realize now that to a large degree, I was just going through the motions. I wasn't ready to fully embody this work yet.

HeartMath techniques seemed so simple yet a part of me was unsure if I was using the tools properly. I questioned whether it was working. I think I was just so stuck in my suffering that change wasn't happening quick enough, and I wanted some relief as soon as possible. Still, I kept at it and found that I could use HeartMath tools to help calm myself down when I was anxious.

Around 2011, I became inspired to put in more of an effort and practiced more of what I would consider classic HeartMath techniques using the technology.

HeartMath technology provides you the opportunity to practice creating heart and brain coherence while simultaneously tracking your progress and giving you feedback. To challenge yourself, there are progressive levels of difficulty within the programs and app. At the easiest challenge levels, reaching coherence through visualization and breathwork is fairly easy. At the more difficult levels, the only way to create and sustain a high level of coherence is by generating and feeling, positive renewing emotions.

After a few months of practicing with the HeartMath technology again, I became very good at achieving high coherence at the lower challenge levels, but I was stuck when it came to the harder levels. The frustration of not getting into coherence at the higher levels was actually negating any positive effects I was experiencing from the previous work. None of the more common visualizations I used were resulting in a coherent state. I tried visualizing beaches, clouds, mountains and anything else that I thought would relax me. I wasn't able to feel the emotion, nothing seemed to be working for me and I was losing my motivation to continue practicing.

Thankfully, I didn't give up! One day, as I was sitting on my bed practicing, I felt a lot of frustration because I was unable to reach coherence on one of the higher challenge levels. I recall sitting on my bed feeling these dense emotions, when suddenly I had a vision of my daughter jumping into my arms and giving me a big hug. My energy shifted instantly! I could feel the hug as if it were actually happening. First, I felt this incredible freedom. I don't know how else to explain it. I just felt free. Then I felt very relaxed, uplifted, energized and focused. Just to confirm what I already knew, the technology made the high-pitched '*ding*,' indicating I had entered high coherence.

This one episode gave me hope. It was a really big moment. I knew, without a doubt, that there was a distinct feeling of coherence which was much different than 'normal.' It was a different state. I felt like I proved to myself that it existed. It also gave me confidence that I could train myself to be in a coherent state. I had just seen the proof. That one experience was beautiful foreshadowing about how valuable this tool was going to be for me in both my personal and professional life.

Over the next several years I implemented the HeartMath biofeedback technology in my office. While it became more common to have conversations about breathwork and regulating an emotional response, I wasn't yet consistent at implementing HeartMath protocols in all my care plans.

At my first Dr. Joe retreat in 2016, he talked about heart coherence and spent a significant amount of time explaining his involvement with research that also happened to include the HeartMath Institute. The foundational principles of coherence, energy, vibration and the quantum field presented in Dr. Joe's work utilize and expand upon the core research done by HeartMath.

The first time I heard Dr. Joe discuss the importance of HeartMath's work around coherence, I felt a wonderful sense of validation. The research Dr. Joe was doing was empowering. Not only was he exploring fascinating concepts, but his work was also validating therapeutic outcomes. I now felt that my prior experience with HeartMath was a huge benefit and I felt a sense of optimism when HeartMath re-entered my consciousness.

HeartMath practices became a much larger part of my life at home and at my office. I started talking about it more with patients and set up a quiet area in my clinic for people to practice the technique. Most importantly, I started using it myself every day.

My belief in the power and effectiveness of the HeartMath techniques grew stronger and I understood the potential game-changing effects of integrating them into my life. By the time the summer of 2019 rolled around, it felt completely natural to finally get certified in clinical applications of the HeartMath techniques and technology, and devote more of my time to teaching and diving deeper into all aspects of the concept of coherence.

The certification course took several months to complete and then I spent an additional several months working on a case study to complete my certification. Not only had my understanding deepened, but I could tell that I would begin to fully implement HeartMath techniques in my patient care programs.

Over the next several months I experimented with different teaching approaches and was eager to continue my learning. In January of 2020 I saw a Facebook post describing an online HeartMath course being offered to the public. I almost skipped it, but as I was scrolling by, I noticed that the program was also open to certified HeartMath professionals. Without knowing anything about the course or who was delivering it, I registered, thinking this was a great opportunity to learn from someone who had years of experience teaching the techniques.

The online course was perfect. There were 4 classes, each between 90 minutes and 2 hours. As advertised, it was for beginners, which allowed me to hear the material being taught in a much different way than the course I took for professionals. I enjoyed the course and was even more motivated to utilize the HeartMath system in my practice. I began to think of additional ways to teach it.

During the first module, I met the instructor, Bruce Cryer, who shared a little bit of his background and involvement with HeartMath. Having been delivering HeartMath programs around the world for more than 25 years, it was evident he knew what he was talking about. I connected with his easygoing approach and teaching style. There was a lightness and humor that accompanied his material. I witnessed his natural ability to connect with people in a loving, heart-centered manner. When Bruce offered to have a follow-up call with any of the professionals taking his course, I jumped at the opportunity to pick his brain a little bit more. Unbeknownst to me, the intuitive sense that led me to initially sign up for the course had been about something much bigger than I expected.

The first private call we had together really changed everything. As it turned out, Bruce Cryer had been the CEO of HeartMath for many years. He was one of a team of people who worked with the founder to create the techniques. He helped build the business in the 1990s and 2000s. I learned that he had a background in theatre, even starring in New York in *The Fantasticks*, the world's longest-running musical, as a young adult, and that dance and music were in his soul.

The conversation went really well, and it led to several others. It was rewarding to find someone who spoke the same language (heart-centered emotions), helped to pioneer the concept of coherence, and had vast experience building and operating a global business. On top of it all, it was so easy to bond with him.

It became obvious that Bruce would make the perfect partner for my wife Aviva and me. We are grateful that Bruce felt the same way and saw our vision. We all share a passion for creating a joyous, inspired life and our unique personalities and strengths fit together very well. Right from the beginning, the *Coherence Revolution* felt coherent.

Although the *Coherence Revolution* expands beyond heart / brain coherence, the education I've had through studying the HeartMath system has been foundational. Their research and technology helped me understand the importance and impact of *love* on an individual's health and relationships.

HeartMath research has shown that experiencing, developing and practicing emotions such as love, gratitude, appreciation and care can become a habit. They've shown that the more you consciously choose to practice an emotion, the easier it will become to feel that emotion. As Bruce says, 'Life becomes so much richer when we allow ourselves to feel deep emotions. What a magnificent human experience it is to FEEL!'

HeartMath techniques are some of the most powerful, efficient and effective tools for sustaining happiness and maintaining the perspective that you have created a life you can be proud of.

Chapter 12

HEART / BRAIN

Heart coherence

Through groundbreaking research, the HeartMath Institute discovered the powerful blend of practicing emotions, specific breathwork and visualizations as a formula to create a coherent heart rhythm and increasing levels of coherence in your life in general. It goes without

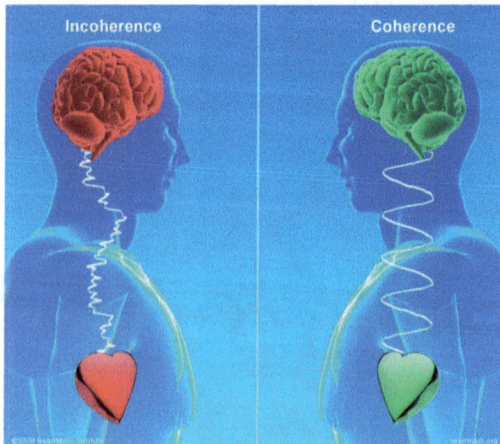

Image courtesy of the HeartMath® Institute – www.heartmath.org

saying that breathing is important to our survival. No matter who you are or how old you are, you understand that in some way, the air you breathe gives you life.

Your breathing rate and heart rate are intricately connected. When you take a breath in, your heart rate goes up; and when you release the breath, your heart rate will go down.

The autonomic nervous system is a complex system which allows your brain to manage about 90% of the processes in your body without having to engage with it consciously. It all happens automatically, beneath the conscious mind. This is the domain of the subconscious mind.

The autonomic nervous system is divided into two branches: the sympathetic and parasympathetic nervous system. The sympathetic nervous system is responsible for your ability to be alert and awake, and it also mediates the stress response, otherwise known as fight or flight (see Appendix).

When the fight-or-flight response is triggered during stressful situations, your heart rate increases to facilitate more blood flow and oxygen to your muscles. When a stressful event passes and your breathing rate slows down, the brain interprets the slowed rhythm as a sign that you are safe. In response, the nervous system relaxes and the stress response dissipates. This primitive response was designed to protect you from any perceived danger. For example, if you were being chased by a bear, your sympathetic nervous system would speed up your heart rate and direct as much blood flow as possible to your big muscles in preparation for you to run away and flee. Additionally, your digestive system, immune system, urinary tract and reproductive systems would all shut down to conserve energy.

Unfortunately, for most people, perceived danger now presents itself in many forms other than physical harm. Accumulated stress from your job, family, or any other circumstance that you feel causes stress, will trigger the fight-or-flight response. Chronic negative thinking and exposure to stressful environments create unhealthy neural programs which are running all the time. Eventually the stress response can be triggered easily by any of your subconscious fears, insecurities and worries instead of the life-threatening circumstances the primal response was supposed to protect you from. As Dr. Joe convincingly states, 'Too often, our future is determined by the stress physiology of our past.'

The parasympathetic nervous system is vital to allowing our system to balance out and reset during acute or prolonged stress. It's activated on exhalation and plays a vital role in resting and digesting as well as repair and healing.

When your body is in a state of coherence, you easily adapt as necessary to your external and internal environments. As stressful events occur, both your heart and brain will adapt to make sure that the appropriate systems in your body have enough blood and oxygen to handle the stressful event and regain balance once it's over.

When you learn how to consciously control your breathing rhythm, you develop the ability to regulate both aspects of your nervous system. By using breathwork and emotional self-regulation tools such as HeartMath, you can learn how to increase your state of coherence and consciously change your physiological state.

Heart focus

One of the simplest yet fundamental tools I use throughout my entire day is heart focus. The concept is to train yourself to automatically focus your attention on your heart any time you have a free moment. Where your attention goes, your energy flows.

Focusing your attention on your heart has many benefits. It grounds you and connects you back to the present moment. It also helps shift your focus and attention away from a racing mind and the outside world. From a practical perspective, it's much easier to change your breathing rhythm when you focus on your heart.

Chapter 13

SUBCONSCIOUS COHERENCE

Subconscious coherence can be defined as the state of mind and body that results from having subconscious beliefs that are congruent with your conscious intentions and goals.

Before learning how to create coherence in any type of conscious way, it's important to understand the impact incoherent subconscious beliefs have on your thoughts, behaviors and emotions. If you are like most people, you will not accomplish your goals if there are constant disagreements between your conscious and subconscious brain.

*In*coherence

One of the largest sources of stress accumulation in your brain is from the incoherent patterns created by conscious and subconscious beliefs that do not match.

Your inner world always tries to make sense of your outer world. Your subconscious mind can make some pretty big assumptions when there is fear, anger or uncertainty towards the external circumstance. The stories you tell yourself are interpreted as fact by your mind.

The emotional response that results from your perception of an event and the story you create ultimately becomes an ingrained neurological pattern and subconscious belief.

When subconscious beliefs are not congruent with your conscious belief patterns and when the vibrational signature of the beliefs don't match, an incoherent wave pattern is created and affects all other coherent rhythms in the body.

Are you creating hardwired triggers?

Sometimes there are situations or events that create such huge emotionally charged responses that they instantly become hardwired in your brain. Your brain holds memories of every event that has happened in your life. Each of those memories also has an associated emotional response. The strength of the memory depends on how strong your emotional connection is to it. When the original event is significant enough, it will be imprinted in areas of the brain, such as the Amygdala (see Appendix), and the neural firing pattern will gain strength every time the mind relives it. When the memory of an event is repeated often enough, eventually a stress response can be triggered simply by subtle cues or reminders from the actual event.

Let me give you a good example. When I was going through a divorce in 2011, it was common to receive numerous e-mails from a lawyer every day. The e-mails were never good. They either had to do with the children or the finances and most times, both.

My body was quickly conditioned to have an anxiety response with each e-mail notification I received. The whole scenario was magnified due to the sophistication of my phone. There were several stages that had the potential to trigger a response. When I received an e-mail, my phone would sound an alert. When I opened my phone, I could see how many e-mails were unread. When I opened the e-mail app I would see all the e-mails in the inbox. Each step was anxiety provoking. When I finally read the contents of any e-mail from the lawyer, I would proceed to have an extended panic attack that could last minutes or the entire day, depending on the severity of the issue.

After a few months, the process had simplified significantly. Due to constant repetition, my body was primed, and it took less and less to trigger a stress response. Eventually every e-mail alert could trigger an anxiety attack. I had been conditioned to respond to an auditory cue.

Thankfully, as I became more aware of the program, I was able to consciously adapt my emotional response to the trigger, and over time developed the ability to dissipate the response quickly.

Is your subconscious preventing you from being coherent?

What is keeping you incoherent? As a health practitioner and someone who has searched for answers my whole adult life, I am no longer surprised by how much we self-sabotage.

Any time there is a subconscious belief system that contradicts your conscious goals or intentions, your chance of success is small. Subconscious programming is extremely strong and determines much of your behavior. The subconscious mind is inextricably linked to the autonomic nervous system, so a subconscious pattern will trigger a stress response based on past experience and belief.

Subconscious beliefs can hold you back for many years and often lead people to engage in destructive activities, thoughts or behaviors that become habits and hardwired patterns. If you find yourself fighting an uphill battle, even when you've made a sincere effort to change, it can be very eye opening to ask yourself, 'What about this destructive activity benefits me?' It seems like a simple question, but it is not.

Imagine sitting in a therapist's office and being asked, 'How does being depressed benefit you?' Your first instinct may be to tell your therapist that it was an insensitive question and that feeling depressed doesn't help you in any way. Some people may even perceive blame within the question itself that can trigger an anxiety attack.

In this scenario, however, it's not about blame. I am not talking about conscious beliefs. There are subconscious programs that are running behind the scenes at all times, kept locked in time by being stuck in stress physiology.

I worked with a patient whose situation illustrated this concept well. Upon asking him what benefits he received from being depressed, he looked confused and quickly realized he did not have a suitable answer.

I knew it was a perfect situation to see what we could discover through the use of muscle testing. I spent a few minutes probing his subconscious mind with questions to determine his belief systems.

The results were fascinating. It seemed that during his depression, the only joy he experienced was when he watched movies. It was something he truly loved. In fact, while he was depressed he was resistant to leaving his home for any reason. He spent the majority of his days watching movies.

This went on for many months and eventually led to the development of a subconscious belief that if he stopped being depressed, he would also have to stop watching movies. He knew he would have to get a job and engage in life. Watching movies was one of the only things in life he enjoyed, so subconsciously, he did everything he could to make that happen.

Another really good example of this was a woman who asked me for help because she was frustrated with her inability to lose weight. She spent many months putting in a sincere effort. She exercised daily and ate really well, yet she was unsuccessful at losing weight. Through the use of muscle testing and a short discussion, her story became clear.

During her daily lunch break, she and her best friend met for coffee and a muffin. She knew that it wasn't helping her diet, but they had been meeting for several years and it had become a regular habit. Her subconscious developed a belief that if she stopped getting the coffee and muffin, she would lose her best friend. Her subconscious made the connection that losing weight was the equivalent of losing a friend. Therefore, she had not lost any weight.

Although it isn't always that easy or obvious, using techniques such as PSYCH-K may help you find subconscious belief systems that are reinforcing beliefs that don't serve you.

Aligning your subconscious and conscious beliefs increases your chance of accomplishing your goal and creates a sense of ease or flow to the process. By eliminating the beliefs that are holding you back, your perception of the situation and the world around you will completely change. Issues that feel like uphill battles start to diminish or disappear, and you begin to see and feel the benefits of all your efforts.

There are many effective methods that can be used to reprogram unwanted subconscious beliefs and reinforce positive ones. There are sophisticated techniques such as Emotional Freedom Technique and PSYCH-K as well as technologies such as BrainTap and Guided Meditation. One of the most common habits to help create positive subconscious beliefs is the use of positive affirmations. It is a simple tool that can be beneficial when used consistently with intention and awareness.

The moment you change your perception is the moment you rewrite the chemistry in your body.
— **Dr. Bruce Lipton**

Muscle testing

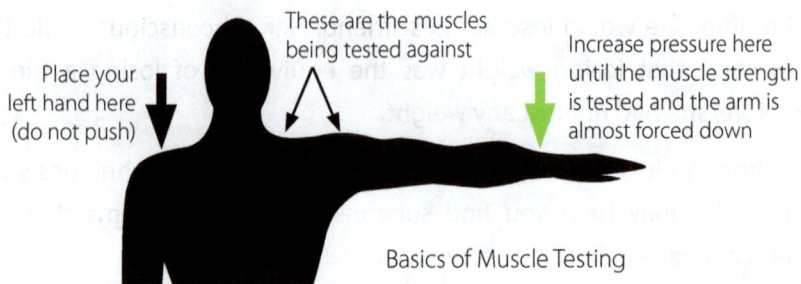

These are the muscles being tested against

Place your left hand here (do not push)

Increase pressure here until the muscle strength is tested and the arm is almost forced down

Basics of Muscle Testing

The technique I describe is a very basic, simplified version but it effectively demonstrates the connection between the conscious and subconscious mind. I encourage you to use these simple instructions to try it for yourself.

What you will find is that when you are thinking positive thoughts or your subconscious is in agreement with a statement, you will feel strong and you will easily keep your arm horizontal to the ground. However, when you think a negative thought or your subconscious is not in agreement with your conscious mind, you will not be able to keep your arm up. Your muscles will not fire properly and you will feel weak.

Go ahead and try it. Have someone try and push your arm down gently while you think about something you really love. After that, do it again while thinking about something really negative in your life. Could you hold your arm up during the negative? Nope? I thought so.

The phenomenon effectively demonstrates that your entire motor nervous system can be impacted by your thoughts alone. Your muscles cannot function properly when there is a disagreement between your conscious and subconscious mind.

It's important to note that although it is common to use the arm as a lever to muscle test, you can test any muscle in the body and the exact same thing will occur. If the muscle you test is the arm and it's weak, the same will hold true for the fingers, legs and back muscles. The reason the arm is generally used is because it's the easiest lever to test.

The muscle weakness that occurs due to negative self-talk or subconscious belief systems has very practical ramifications for people in their day-to-day lives. Whether you sit at your desk, drive your car or stand all day, most people don't spend the day encouraging themselves and repeating positive affirmations. It's much more common to have inner dialogue that is not conducive to creating the healthiest you possible.

It's common to have thoughts such as, 'I'm behind already,' 'I'm tired,' 'I'm bored,' 'I don't like my boss,' 'I hate this job,' 'I still have to do laundry and get groceries,' 'I'm exhausted.' The negative commentary can carry on all day.

Remember what happened to your arm strength when you muscle tested for negative stressful situations – it weakened. That's exactly what happens when you engage in negative self-talk all day. Your muscles stop firing properly and perform as if they are weak. Every muscle in your body will stop firing properly.

This is significant because the muscles, which are designed to protect and support your spine as well as oppose gravity, won't do their job effectively. It results in an incredible amount of force and excessive wear and tear on your spine.

A basic understanding of anatomy sheds light on how the health of your spine directly impacts the health of your entire nervous system. The spine is made of bone, which is the hardest substance in your body. It's essentially an armor. It protects the most delicate tissues, your brain and spinal cord. If the armor is damaged, the tissue it is protecting will also be more vulnerable.

Once you understand this, it is easy to see how incoherent thoughts can directly lead to just about all of the common health issues people deal with, including digestive upset, chronic fatigue, back pain, headaches and a weakened ability to deal with sickness and disease.

Random negative thoughts

Do you ever find yourself having mean, rude or even insulting thoughts towards other people? Do you have thoughts that scare you or trigger guilt just because you've had them? Have you ever asked yourself if your thoughts were true?

When your brain is under stress and your fear pathways fire on overdrive, the judgmental aspect of the conscious brain does not always fire coherently. Therefore, the thoughts that are produced are a direct result of the amount of stress your brain is under. Inappropriate, negative subconscious beliefs may race through your mind or thoughts that may have nothing to do with your actual belief system. The negative thoughts are just that...thoughts.

Although it may be disturbing to have these thoughts about other people, or even yourself, a part of your mind, usually the ego, fires off fearful, negative and what it thinks are protective thoughts. When you feel hurt by someone emotionally and experience a stress response, automatic negative thoughts are the brain's attempt to protect you from any perceived danger.

If you felt deserted by someone, perhaps a negative thought would be triggered that said, 'I don't like them anyways,' or 'I hope they get fired,' or something that is equally as mean.

These negative thoughts are an incoherent response to an incoherent situation, which is actually an attempt by the brain to create more coherence. Unfortunately, you cannot attain coherence through a fearful, defensive act.

I often felt distressed if I had demeaning or awful thoughts about myself or others. There were statements or words I used in my mind that were disturbing to me. I knew those thoughts were not an accurate portrayal of how I truly felt.

Thoughts can make us sick

There is a direct link between the thoughts you think and your body's ability to heal and maintain your health.

Each time you have a thought, an emotion is elicited that initiates chemical reactions primarily in your brain, heart and adrenal glands. The strength of these reactions depends on your perception and interpretation of the event.

If negative emotions are produced, the chemicals produced are depleting in nature, which means proper cell function will be impaired and your body will utilize energy inefficiently, leading to exhaustion and dysfunction. It can be said then that your body will literally function with less ease or in a state of dis-ease.

If your body functions in a state of dis-ease for long periods of time, eventually the dysfunction will reach a point when it will be called an actual disease. You can make yourself sick simply by the thoughts you think.

Many people do just that. They spend all day thinking incoherently and then wonder why they feel so terrible and struggle to maintain their health.

Being conditioned to create incoherence

Dr. Joe Dispenza's book, *Breaking the Habit of Being Yourself*, discusses the complex chemical reactions and different physiological states that occur in both renewing and depleting emotional states.

Dr. Joe emphasizes and explains that positive, elevated or happy thoughts create chemicals that make you feel good or happy while negative or insecure thoughts produce chemicals that make you feel exactly the way you are thinking. Every chemical that is released in the brain is literally a messenger that informs and instructs the physical body. That is how the body begins to feel the way the mind is thinking.

This type of conditioning works for both uplifting and stressful circumstances. If a thought produces a chemical and a chemical produces an emotion, then every time you produce the same thought, you will produce the same chemical and, therefore, the same emotion.

If you think a thought repeatedly and produce the same chemical enough times, it becomes a habit. The body literally develops a need for the chemical. As the need becomes hardwired, the body becomes addicted to the response and craves the chemical before it's even been created.

The body's need for the stress hormones will actually stimulate the mind to create the appropriate fearful or depleting thought so the stress response will be triggered. Over time, the feeling and emotion can start to happen even before the thought. Eventually the brain doesn't care if the thought (stimulus) is there anymore; it just wants the adrenal rush and the flow of chemicals that satiate the brain.

Adrenaline and the other stress hormones are strong nervous system stimulants. The cravings your body develops for stress hormones are similar to that for caffeine and nicotine in coffee and cigarettes respectively. Your brain habitually triggers the release of the stress hormones and your body suffers because of it.

Addiction to anxiety

I'd like to expand further on being conditioned for specific emotions. In my case, I didn't feel many emotions. My emotions were always expressed as anxiety.

Anxiety is both a state of mind and body. When you are anxious, your mind produces incoherent thoughts and triggers the release of the hormones and chemicals of stress. Over time, and with repetition, your brain becomes very efficient at producing those chemicals. The production of stress hormones becomes habitual, and your body not only expects them but eventually begins to crave them.

Your body craves the chemicals of stress and eventually develops an addiction to anxiety.

This is one of those concepts that just knocked me over when I heard it. I remember sitting in one of Dr. Joe's lectures, and as I was listening to him explain this concept, my perception of my past and present reality changed. The voice inside my head was literally screaming, 'My body is addicted to the chemicals of stress!' It was a eureka moment.

As Bruce Lipton talks about in *The Biology of Belief*, you subconsciously plan and seek out additional stressful situations to occur so that your body will produce the specific stress hormones that you are craving.

Once you understand this concept, you can begin to change.

All the responses you have to the people, places, situations or things in your life are based on a neural program created from past experiences, from the stress physiology of your past. Once you become conscious of the program, you have an opportunity to create a new program, a new pattern and eventually a new reality.

If you think about a typical habit or even an addiction you have in your life, you will notice a few similarities. First, you can't picture doing the habit any other way. Second, you accomplish the habit as the result of a subconscious program you barely realize is happening. Third, your body wants to keep doing the same habit. The more you do it, the more natural it feels and the more the habit becomes ingrained in your subconscious.

The same three elements can be applied to the process of anxiety and stress. Once anxiety becomes an addiction, the mind will continue to search for and create additional anxiety-producing situations to replace the one that you've just solved. It can seem like there is one huge problem after the next.

When anxiety becomes the nervous system's set point, the mind's goal is to elicit another stress response. Your mind will ensure that the body has plenty of opportunities to practice and it essentially becomes effective at producing the hormones of stress.

Think about a habit you've been unable to change. If you're used to living a sedentary lifestyle, think about the amount of energy and effort required to do a yoga class or start an exercise program. Although you know it will feel good and you know how healthy it is for you, it will still take a lot of mental energy and a huge effort to succeed at changing your habitual pattern.

If you're like most people, change is hard because you have so many habits, addictions and hardwired neural programs you're not even aware of. Have you ever noticed that you wash and dry your body in the exact same pattern after every shower? Have you ever driven home and had zero recollection of the left-hand turn you made onto your street? Both are examples of subconscious hardwired programming. They're habits. Try switching it up. Make a conscious effort to wash and dry yourself in a different order or take an alternate route home from work. See how it feels. Most likely, it will feel bizarre and require a little more conscious energy and focus to break the programming.

Anxiety is no different. It's a hardwired neural program that requires conscious effort to create new chemicals and new emotions to replace the habitual ones.

Imagine the amount of energy it would take for you to force a smile when you are anxious and stressed out? Although it can seem impossible to initiate, it quickly gets easier because when you smile, the muscles used to perform the action stimulate the brain to produce the chemicals of joy and happiness. The chemical production is directly connected to the contraction of the facial muscles.

Smiling into a mirror seems easy enough, but in reality, if you're feeling depleting emotions such as anger, depression or anxiety, it won't come easy. When your default emotions are depleting and incoherent, it requires the conscious creation of renewing emotions to change your habitual programming. If you make the conscious choice to smile, you are capable of breaking the pattern. It's like anything else: the more you practice, the easier it gets.

It is extremely helpful to practice habits like this because every time you produce the chemicals of joy rather than the chemicals of stress, the new neural programs will be reinforced. The more things you do in your life that lead to joy and happiness, the more often you counteract your addiction to anxiety.

In other words, with enough practice and effort, your body will learn how to mitigate and eliminate the stress response. You can become very proficient at consciously creating the release of positive and happy chemicals in your brain.

When you practice creating positive emotions such as joy, happiness, excitement, passion, relaxation, calm, relief and peace, your perception of the world around you begins to shift. You will start to see possibilities. You simply react differently and begin to create new patterns.

Thankfully, the same concepts that make it possible for thoughts to be so depleting, can also enable you to use your thoughts to create inspiration, joy and happiness. When your thoughts are positive and uplifting, your cells utilize energy more efficiently, your systems function in harmony with each other and you are connected to your innate intelligence.

Chapter 14

EMOTIONAL COHERENCE

―――――――――

Emotional coherence can be defined as your body's ability to create a situationally appropriate emotional response that encourages a renewal of your emotional system rather than one of depletion and overwhelm.

―――――――――

Throughout your life, you experience many types of situations that require a wide range of emotional responses. The greater your awareness and ability to access your entire emotional landscape, the easier you will adapt to any circumstance.

Most people find themselves having incoherent emotional responses throughout their day on a regular basis. A typical scenario of being stuck in bumper-to-bumper traffic can produce a massive stress response.

While that situation wouldn't pose any real threat, if you feel frustrated and out of control when you are delayed in traffic, the anxiety that is triggered can feel just as severe as any other stressful or difficult circumstance.

Habits and neurological patterns are created in your life when you engage in repetitive activities. The vast majority of your thoughts, actions and behaviors are repeated subconsciously every day. Perhaps the most repetitive thing we do every day is think, and each thought has the ability to produce an emotion. By repeating the same thoughts on a daily basis, it becomes a practice. It is then logical to conclude that we are basically practicing our emotions every day.

The more often you feel a specific emotion, especially a strong one, the quicker and easier it becomes to produce it again. Sometimes, if the pattern is hardwired, the emotion seems to appear instantaneously or even before the thought.

Try to think of someone who pushes your buttons and frustrates you every time they behave a certain way. By having the same reaction to them repeatedly, your response becomes an ingrained habit. A neural circuit is created in your brain, and it becomes easier and easier to feel frustrated by that person.

If that is truly the case, doesn't it make sense to practice appropriate emotions for each circumstance or occasion that challenges your ability to evoke renewing emotions? What if you spent the entire time you were stuck in traffic consciously finding ways to laugh or learn something? Are you willing to practice the emotions of your ideal response to any situation? The more familiar an emotion feels, the easier it is to create.

While we don't want to experience chronic depleting emotions, sometimes dense emotions are necessary as we navigate life. Choosing the proper emotions to practice becomes even more important when your thoughts are incoherent. For example, if someone passes away, adding coherence to your nervous system will help facilitate a healthy and natural grieving process that eventually results in a renewal of your emotional energy. Practicing emotions such as gratitude, peace or calm would be far more appropriate than perhaps happiness or joy.

Renewing emotions can be both high and low energy. They can be elevated and energetic such as joy or excitement, and they can also be more subdued such as tranquil or peaceful.

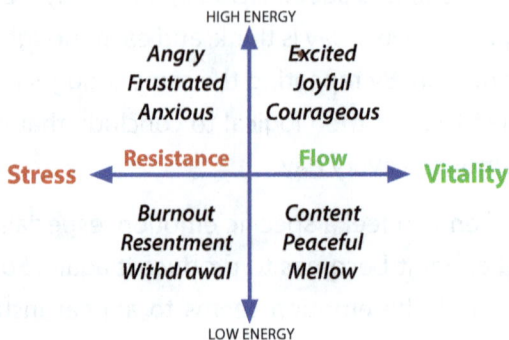

HIGH ENERGY

Angry   Excited
Frustrated   Joyful
Anxious   Courageous

Resistance   Flow

Stress ◄——————► Vitality

Burnout   Content
Resentment   Peaceful
Withdrawal   Mellow

LOW ENERGY

Circumstances usually dictate which emotion is most appropriate. For instance, it may not be ideal to arrive at a friend's party in a tranquil, serene mood if everyone else is exuberant and full of high energy. The opposite also holds true. If you are invited over to a friend's place to relax and share a good conversation, being energetic and ready to dance may not be ideal.

We all have the innate ability to regulate our emotions. The more we practice a wide variety of emotions, the better we are at responding and adapting to those emotions. When you practice emotions such as peace or calm, the nervous system relaxes and requires less energy. When you practice emotions such as excitement and joy, your body releases energy to perpetuate and fuel that emotional response. You can use your understanding of renewing emotional states to choose between a high or low energy response.

Practicing your future

When you relive a situation in your mind and feel the associated emotion, your brain believes it's happening all over again. Your brain won't distinguish whether it's only happening internally, in your mind, or externally, in reality. The same reasoning will hold true for practicing the emotions of your future. Eventually it will become easier and easier to elicit your chosen future emotional state.

As you practice, your brain will begin to believe and respond as if your future is happening now. Not only will it seem more possible to attain, but the chances of it occurring greatly increase. The more you live your life as if it is exactly the way you want it, the easier it is to believe it's going to happen. It becomes more familiar to you.

Your senses are also crucial to this process because they are the interface between your inner and outer world and can be used to practice evoking and strengthening specific emotions. The likelihood of manifesting your dream life is infinitely greater when you strengthen your emotional attachment to it and make the possibility of it feel as real as possible. Using each of your senses to magnify your emotional response will help strengthen your chances of reaching your goal.

Let's say, for example, your goal is to create coherence in a relationship. As you practice visualizing your optimal relationship, your senses can be used to increase positive emotional responses.

If you reflect on the questions below, your answers will help strengthen your ability to create an emotional connection to the visualization.

What types of things would you like to see when you create your ideal relationship? Does it calm you to visualize taking a walk in nature together? Do you enjoy staring across the table at your partner? Do you have memories of watching the sunset or looking into each other's eyes? Do you see specific places where you enjoy spending time together?

What types of smells would elicit loving emotions or relaxed moods? What does a romantic dinner taste like to you?

When you close your eyes, can you feel yourself taking your partner's hand while on a walk? Can you elicit a positive emotion by imagining yourself dancing together? Do you enjoy listening to birds sing in your backyard? What types of music do you enjoy listening together?

Each sense increases your emotional connection to your future reality.

How to practice an emotion

Perhaps the most important concept and the very heart of the book and live course, *Coherence Revolution*, is the magic of consciously eliciting and practicing renewing emotions. As you create your own *Coherence Revolution*, you will learn how to gain conscious control over your emotions through the creation of a personalized and powerful daily practice.

You will effectively learn to regulate your emotions through the use of HeartMath techniques, your senses, the words you say, the thoughts you think and the natural world around you.

As you engage in the process, I encourage you to literally pick a renewing, calming or uplifting emotion and practice it. Do this as often as you can, anytime and anywhere.

Practicing positive emotions can be a bit intimidating if you aren't in the habit of feeling them. It is best to start with a gentle emotion such as calm instead of stronger emotions such as peace or tranquility. In much the same way, it is also easier to practice feeling uplifted or joyful than it is to practice emotions such as passion or excitement. Start easy and then challenge yourself.

When I started practicing emotions, I found that the easiest emotion for me to practice was relief. I had a strong memory that made it an easy emotion to recall. When I closed my eyes, I remembered receiving my grades from board exams I wrote all the way back in 1996. I could still feel the weight of the package in my hands before I opened it. I could hear the rip of the envelope and I could feel the genuine relief I felt when I saw the capital A with a circle around it at the top of the exam as I pulled it out. Any time I wanted to practice that feeling I could close my eyes and recreate the same scenario.

The board exam scenario is a good example of using multiple senses to increase the effectiveness of the visualization. The smell of muffins always accompanies the thought of opening the envelope. That seems quite random, right? Well, I opened the envelope in the kitchen and at the time, there were muffins baking in the oven. Now when I remember the event, I smell the muffins. It's not even the real smell. It's my memory of being in the kitchen smelling the muffins. The memory of the smell strengthens the feeling of relief because it makes the visualization more vivid and real. It provides another layer of emotional connection.

In the complete visualization, I can clearly hear my mom congratulating me and I can feel her giving me a loving hug. Not only does that address the auditory component but it utilizes the sense of touch which is also immensely powerful.

Another way to practice an emotion is to actually practice saying specific words with greater intention and energy. Just like smiling in the mirror helps release more chemicals of joy, saying specific words out loud reinforces and elicits a wide variety of emotions.

As I have discussed, I use a technique called Ho'oponopono. Using the technique is extremely simple and involves repeating the phrases, 'Thank you,''I love you,''Forgive me,''I am sorry.'

Each of these words and phrases has their own meaning, vibration and can elicit specific emotions.

For example, when I feel like my heart is closed, I repeat the phrase, 'I love you.'

As I put in a genuine effort and start to think of areas in my life to which I would like to apply renewing emotions, it becomes easier to create and feel them.

When I want to feel more gratitude, I simply repeat the phrase, 'Thank you.' It's the feelings that those words trigger that change my physiological state.

By following the process set out in *Coherence Revolution*, you will have the opportunity to explore your senses and discover the most effective way for you to elicit the emotions of your dream life.

Chapter 15

COHERENCE IN YOUR SENSES

Creating coherence using all five senses

If strong emotions can be triggered by specific thoughts about an event and over time they develop a hardwired connection to each other, then eventually you will be able to stimulate the specific memory by both a thought and the emotion associated with it. It works both ways. A thought can trigger an emotion, and an emotion can trigger a thought.

We also know that when one of your senses is stimulated, it can awaken an emotional memory and allow you to recall the event or thought process from the past. Commonly, what happens is that one of your senses will be stimulated (auditory, visual, kinesthetic, taste, smell) and trigger an emotional response. When the emotional response is due to a specific memory, the familiarity of the emotional response can actually trigger specific thoughts.

One of the best examples I can think of involves the strong smell of a specific type of gasoline. To this day, when I walk through a few select places near my home, the smell instantly stimulates memories of waiting for the camp bus as an eight-year-old child. Short flashes of past memories and feelings can appear and I feel like a little boy again. For a few brief moments, I can remember the way it felt to be waiting for the bus and even how it felt to hold my lunch box. It all comes rushing back with one smell. That's all it takes to trigger a real and vivid memory.

All five of your senses can elicit strong emotional responses. All of your senses affect the amount of coherence you are able to achieve and maintain. The foods you taste and the sounds you hear can trigger memories and emotions. Certain colours may calm or invigorate you. The texture of fabric and materials you touch can affect your mood. Heat and cold can provide comfort, but if they are too extreme, they can elicit a stress response or cause a state of dis-ease. Each sense has the capability to deplete you or supercharge your ability to gain coherence in every aspect of your life.

KINESTHETIC COHERENCE

―――――――――

Kinesthetic coherence occurs when any physical movement, touch or sensory stimuli increases coherence in any aspect of your being and helps you access renewing emotional states.

―――――――――

What we 'feel' can be interpreted in many different ways. For our purposes, *kinesthetic coherence* refers to your sense of touch and movement of your physical body. What sensations are your nerve fibers detecting on your skin? Do you wear clothing that is soft and cozy or thin and breathable? What messages are your muscles sending to your brain? Do you feel flexible or stiff? Does your body feel strong?

As a brain-based chiropractor, my goal is to help people achieve their optimal state of healing so they can adapt and increase their resilience to stressful situations. I look for ways to help my patients break chronic stress patterns that have developed in their spine and nervous system. Too many people endure long periods in stressful environments each day. It takes a toll. The most common physical stressors that accumulate and deplete your energy involve any and all of the following repetitive activities and actions: sitting, sleeping, standing, walking, exercising, lifting, grabbing, pulling and reaching.

The more efficiently you can adapt to and perform these activities, the easier it is to prevent them from overwhelming you and affecting other aspects of your health.

Although the majority of people seek chiropractic care to alleviate their back pain, the most powerful way I can facilitate a shift towards a more coherent state is with an adjustment.

In much the same way that the research conducted in quantum physics has inspired me, I am excited that there is finally chiropractic research validating a neurological approach to care. One of the most impactful aspects of adjusting the spine is that it is an effective 'neurological interrupt' that can help reset and change chronic neurological patterns.

Unfortunately, there is a lot of misinformation about chiropractors and why spinal care is so important. The goal of chiropractic care is not to simply reduce pain or eliminate symptoms, nor is it meant to treat or cure sickness and disease. The focus of care in my office is to optimize the function of the spine, extremities, and the entire brain and nervous system.

Due to the confusion around chiropractic care, I receive a lot of questions from my patients about

Chiropractic research

The research of Dr. Haavik explores the effects of a chiropractic adjustment on brain function. In particular, she investigates what happens in the brain when a chiropractor adjusts dysfunctional spinal segments. She has utilized sophisticated neuroscience techniques such as somatosensory-evoked electroencephalography and transcranial magnetic brain stimulation to investigate the effects of a chiropractic adjustment on somatosensory processing, sensorimotor integration and motor cortical output.

https://www.heidihaavik.com/pages/research

what conditions I can help them with or if the improvement they saw in their health was due to the care they received. I am often asked if it's possible for chiropractic care to benefit people with digestive disorders. I am approached by people who want to improve the quality of their sleep. Patients want to know if it's possible to feel more relaxed after their adjustment. The answer is always yes.

As a result of acting as a 'neurological interrupt' (see Appendix), a chiropractic adjustment resets and improves the quality of communication with the brain. It will also result in an increase of brain wave frequencies which are healing and renewing in nature. The benefits my patients have seen after receiving care, have reinforced for me that humans are self-healing and self-regulating organisms. Ultimately, it is much easier for your body to maintain a state of health when your nervous system is functioning optimally.

Every millisecond there are millions of messages travelling back and forth between the brain and body through the nervous system. Your fingers relay information such as temperature, pressure and texture, from everything you touch back to the brain. Your feet do the same and they also relay information that is crucial to keeping you balanced and upright. Your hips, knees and shoulder joints convey information about strength and posture, which is necessary to ensure proper movement. Additionally, all areas of your skin relay information to the brain about the textures and sensations you perceive. When the sensory information transmitted to the brain is coherent, the body responds by functioning at its best, utilizing energy efficiently and healing effectively.

Sports / physical challenge

One of the most common ways to experience *kinesthetic coherence* occurs while you are competing or engaged in something physical. Athletes often talk about feeling *'in the zone'* and how their bodies feel balanced and in the flow of the activity they are engaged in. It can be an intoxicating, addictive experience.

Part of your ability to have that type of experience is due to conditioning. It obviously helps to be in the best physical shape possible. Additionally, when you increase your level of expertise and confidence to the point that you can get lost in the moment, exercise can facilitate a spiritual experience. When you feel coherent and *in the zone* during a physical challenge or sport, time tends to stand still and your senses become heightened.

Over the years, I've learned how to create that type of coherent state by engaging in my athletic and physical passions as often as possible.

There are various factors that impact *kinesthetic coherence*. It is helpful to identify all the physical and sensory stressors you are exposed to so that you can make conscious choices based on which ones are renewing and therefore, increase your coherence level throughout your day.

Exercise

When your exercise program is in coherence with your highest good, it will ensure that you are strong and stable. Your body will use energy more efficiently and you will increase your ability to adapt to the strain of daily life.

Although the type of program may vary depending on your personal goals, it is important that the exercise you choose works with your body, not against it. The benefits must outweigh the costs.

In many cases, although your intentions are good, the impact of the exercise you engage in is more detrimental than the perceived or actual benefit you receive. Some people thrive on doing high-impact exercise, while for others, it will overload their body and cause short or even possibly long-term damage. Yoga is another good example. Some classes require advanced balance and flexibility that may be detrimental for people suffering with conditions such as scoliosis, arthritis or any other type of chronic injury. However, for others, the same class may be a fundamental healing practice.

Creating a coherent exercise plan involves understanding several factors. The first question to ask yourself is, 'Am I committed?' In other words, do you have a big enough *why* to motivate you. If you are connected to and passionate about your *why*, the chance of following through is much greater.

Next, it's important that your exercise program addresses your concerns and accomplishes your goals. Are you trying to gain strength, increase flexibility, create stability or improve your cardiovascular function? How do you feel before, during and after the exercise? Are you left exhausted and in pain, or do you feel energized and renewed? Do you enjoy the activity and look forward to it? What is your mindset towards it?

It's also crucial to make sure you have the time to incorporate the exercise you've chosen into your daily routine. One of the biggest challenges even dedicated people face is finding the time to implement their customized exercise program.

To set yourself up for success, it's important to create a plan that is realistic, fits your schedule, addresses your goals and inspires you to consistently take action.

Clothes, jewelry and accessories

The clothing and accessories you wear have direct and indirect effects on how you feel depending on the type of fabrics and materials used and how they fit your body.

What is your preference?

Do you like materials that are thick or thin? Do you like a tight or loose fit? Do you prefer polyester or cotton? Some materials feel heavy, warm and protective while others are more breathable, cool and soft.

When you become conscious and aware of what you choose to wear, you have the opportunity to elicit a strong renewing emotional response based on how your body feels.

Sleep

Since you're most likely going to spend a third of your life in bed, it would be ideal to create healthy habits which support your body and help elevate your state of coherence.

Lying in awkward, twisted positions causes excess wear and tear on your spine. Sleeping in an ergonomic position, on a supportive mattress, with the proper-size pillow, not only alleviates the strain but keeps your airway open so you can breathe easily. We already know how influential your breath can be in creating a coherent mind and body.

As you assess your sleep position and your mattress, pay attention to how you feel during the night as well as in the morning. Reducing the strain on your spine as much as possible can be the difference between waking up in pain and feeling depleted or waking up feeling inspired and energized.

The human touch

Whether it's a handshake, hug, shoulder grab or pat on the back, there are many factors to consider when assessing how coherently you receive someone else's touch. The temperature, the texture, the strength, the size and the rhythm will all contribute to or reduce your state of coherence.

Sitting

The surface you sit on as well as the positioning of your spine will impact your entire body's ability to be in a coherent state. While it is not ideal to spend most of your day sitting, the fact is that sitting is unavoidable. Movement is the key to life, so by its very nature, sitting and being still depletes you.

Humans were never meant to sit in the prolonged postures most of us commonly use. The best way to reduce the negative, depleting effects of sitting is to constantly change your positioning and limit the amount of time you are sedentary.

The surfaces you stand on

Your brain is always seeking balance. The surfaces you stand on impact the sensory feedback between your feet and brain. The brain will make adaptive corrections based on factors such as the texture, density and whether the ground is level. When you have a healthy posture, your spine and extremities are under less physical stress, and this allows you to use your energy efficiently. However, it takes far more effort and energy to operate your body if you have to stand for long periods and endure tilting to one side, balancing on an uneven surface or standing on a hard surface with no shock absorption. One way to minimize the wear and tear on your body is to choose proper and supportive footwear.

Your steering wheel

This is another example of something you may touch several times a day and is particularly important because not only do you feel the material of the steering wheel but the car's vibration is also transmitted through it. When your hands feel good gripping the steering wheel, you can feel like you're the king or queen of the road. If the vibration feels annoying, the leather is fading, there are tears, sticky spots or grinding, the experience of holding the steering wheel becomes depleting and you feel less coherent during and after the drive.

Beverage containers

How many small energy drains do you experience in a day? All of the little annoyances and irritations you experience on a daily basis can accumulate and eventually have an impact on your overall resilience and energy level.

Whether it's your water bottle, coffee or tea mug, smoothie cup or even a recyclable straw, ask yourself how it feels on your lips? Is it heavy or light? Do you enjoy and look forward to the sip or is it constantly leaking and causing you annoyance? Is it too cold or does it burn you? Is the experience a small energy drain or a consistently enjoyable aspect of your day?

Kinesthetic inquiry

Spend some time exploring the types of physical sensations and activities that leave you feeling renewed and energized or relaxed and peaceful. What types of things can you do to increase kinesthetic coherence?

Do you have a preference of tools to use when you're cooking, cutting, chopping?

Do you prefer using wood or metal utensils?

Do you enjoy using your hands to do gardening, pottery or sculpting?

How do your feet feel when you walk in the grass or the sand?

When you shower or bathe, do you prefer the feel of a bar of soap or a sponge against your body?

Do you enjoy gentle movement or vigorous dance?

Once you have had the chance to assess that which depletes or renews you, I encourage you to make choices that will utilize kinesthetic coherence to your advantage.

VISUAL COHERENCE

Visual coherence occurs when any visual stimuli increases coherence in any aspect of your being and helps you access renewing emotional states.

One of the most practical challenges some people face while learning how to benefit from *visual coherence* is their actual vision. People like me who wear glasses or contacts may have additional concerns which may include: colour blindness, headaches, dizziness, nausea and varying degrees of vision loss. There is nothing I am more grateful for than my contact lenses and glasses. I am reminded of how beautiful the world is every time I wake up and put on my glasses or put my contact lenses in.

When you start to delve into *visual coherence*, you will find that different images produce different emotions. Being conscious of what you are looking at throughout your day can have a drastic effect on your overall coherence level. As with all your senses, what your visual field perceives will either renew or deplete you.

In today's world, it's even more important to pay attention to this because most people spend so much time staring at technology and computer screens which can be incredibly depleting.

A quick assessment of the environments you spend most of your time in can shed light on whether your surroundings are a source of inspiration or another means of accumulating stress.

Once you are aware of your visual landscape, you can create different atmospheres based on the type of emotion you would like to evoke. You can surround yourself with consciously chosen plants, decor, renewing images and photographs that elicit positive emotions.

For instance, you may find adding pictures of your family to your office desk will help remind you why you are working so hard. Moving your desk so you have a clear view through the window might change your outlook both literally and figuratively.

The same type of introspection can be used at home. The more strategic you are about placing images or pictures in appropriate areas, the more benefit you will receive.

An additional way to use *visual coherence* to your benefit is wearing colours that help facilitate positive emotions. Colour can also be used throughout your home and all of your personal accessories to impact the way you feel.

Sometimes simply neatening up your space to avoid looking at clutter can change the way you cope with the rest of your day. There are many times though, that visually, authenticity helps. There is nothing more powerful than actually going to a window or outside to spend some time observing nature.

It really is your choice. From the moment you wake up, what are you visually focusing on? You choose what images you spend time viewing both externally and internally. You have the choice to wake up and view an inspiring image or check your Facebook page. You can choose to wear colours that calm or energize you based upon the day you've got planned. You can choose the scenic route on your walk to work or make time at lunch to go sit in the park.

Have fun and enjoy using the visual opportunities you have to increase coherence in every aspect of your life whenever possible.

AUDITORY COHERENCE

Auditory coherence occurs when any sound or frequency stimulates or increases coherence in any aspect of your being and helps you access renewing emotional states.

The human ear can commonly hear frequencies between 20 and 20 000 Hz. There are many factors involved in determining how coherent an auditory frequency is for you: the pitch, tone, note, rhythm and volume. This applies to the human voice, music, technology, nature and any other sound frequency your ears perceive. When a sound feels coherent, you can feel it throughout your entire body. Depending on the type of auditory frequencies you are exposed to, a wide range of emotional responses are possible.

There are many sources for the different sounds and frequencies that our auditory system processes. All sounds have the potential to deplete or renew us. Most people intuitively know that listening to the sound of waves or birds stimulates a relaxing response in the brain. Conversely, the sound of traffic or a chaotic environment will induce an incoherent stress response.

Music can have an enormous influence on brain function which differs for each individual based on what resonates with them. Variations in genres and types of music can produce an array of emotional reactions. While classical music provides a way for some people to relax and unwind, others resonate more with jazz or country. It can be the interpretation of words from a song that evokes an emotion, or simply the tone or melody.

There are many different naturally occurring frequencies to which our brains resonate. These frequencies help us attain specific physiological states. With a quick search on YouTube, you can find some examples of healing frequencies.

_____

Examples of sound frequencies influencing our brain and nervous system

- *Alpha waves.* Recent research suggests the stimulation of alpha brainwaves may help you become more creative and possibly even help treat depression. The electrical pulses produced from masses of neurons communicating with each other form wave-like patterns – hence the term brainwave.
  (https://www.caba.org.uk/help-and-guides/information/how-and-why-boost-your-alpha-brainwaves)

- *Theta waves.* Some of the reported benefits of listening to theta waves immersed in meditative audio tracks are easier meditation practice, increased levels of creativity, body healing and rejuvenation, increased mental clarity, lucid dreaming, increased vigor, improved relationships, ability to tap into your conscious mind, better sleep.
  (https://www.binauralbeatsfreak.com/brainwave-entrainment/the-benefits-of-theta-binaural-beats)

- *Schumann Resonance.* 'At any given moment, about 2,000 thunderstorms roll over Earth, producing some 50 flashes of lightning every second. Each lightning burst creates electromagnetic waves that begin to circle around Earth captured between Earth's surface and a boundary about 60 miles up. Some of the waves – if they have just the right wavelength – combine, increasing in strength, to create a repeating atmospheric heartbeat known as Schumann resonance.' (NASA)

Being out of sync with the Schumann resonance (Earth's heartbeat) can be depleting and can lead to health concerns such as anxiety, insomnia, illness and a suppressed immune system. Conversely, when we are in sync with the Earth's heartbeat, the body is able to heal and renew itself.

- The 396 Hz frequencies for liberating one from fear and guilt,

- The 417 Hz frequencies for facilitating change and undoing situations,

- The 528 Hz frequencies for miracles and transformations like DNA repair,

- The 639 Hz frequencies for relationships and reconnecting,

- The 741 Hz frequencies for getting solutions and expressing themselves,

- The 852 Hz frequencies for returning one to a spiritual order (https://naturehealingsociety.com/solfeggio/).

A great example of a specific frequency are *Schumann waves*. As you listen to audio files that use these waves, your brain entrains to the specific frequency and helps you to feel grounded.

Sound can be used in many ways to improve health and create increased coherence in the body. The words we hear, the music we listen to and the natural sounds around us all have the ability to create coherence and renewal or to create contraction and depletion.

As you explore and discover new ways to utilize *auditory coherence*, it's important to assess noise pollution as well as any other agitating sounds you may be exposed to on a daily basis. Do you hear the buzz of electricity in the wires outside your window or do you have the pleasure of listening to the birds singing on a nearby tree? Do you hear people speaking lovingly towards each other, or are you exposed to yelling and arguing at work or at home? Does hearing the nightly news in the background unsettle you? Do you have music playing softly in the background to comfort you? The more aware you become of the auditory frequencies you are exposed to on a daily basis, the more conscious you can be about eliminating the incoherent sounds which can leave you feeling depleted.

An effective way to create a high level of coherence through sound is to combine several auditory approaches. You can create an extremely powerful experience by recording yourself reading positive affirmations at a time when you are feeling uplifted and experiencing a high level of coherence. In future times of need, you'll be able to use your own voice and emotional signature. When you listen back to the recording, you will hear yourself in a more optimal state and can tap into your own power to elevate your vibration and nurture your soul.

There are so many great ways to involve sound in your life: music, meditations, positive affirmations, BrainTap sessions, listening to nature, hearing a calming voice, singing and playing an instrument. Discovering all the ways you can utilize *auditory coherence* can be a very enjoyable process.

The impact of words

The words we use matter. Whether they are said out loud or in your head, words convey specific meanings and vibrate in a wide range of frequencies which can be felt by both the person speaking and the person being spoken to.

Although spoken words are more powerful, even words said silently in your mind have an impact. The intensity may not be as strong but the thought of a word carries the same vibration and intention as saying it out loud.

Negative words have a more powerful impact than positive words on both yourself and others. Words that are perceived as bad, insulting, rude or destructive can elicit strong emotional responses that alter your physiological state very quickly, triggering reactions from your stress physiology and throwing your system out of coherence.

Words can be depleting or renewing depending on their use and their intention. Depleting words drain your energy and can easily affect your mood negatively. Renewing words energize and uplift you. Ultimately, it's your interpretation of the words that provides meaning and therefore, impacts your system. Through that meaning, your body will create an emotional response which results in the production and release of specific chemicals and neurotransmitters in the brain. It's that process of perception followed by the chemical release that will determine if you are happy, sad, energetic, exhausted, healthy or sick.

How mindful are you about the words you use towards yourself or others? Have you ever asked yourself if what you were about to say was good for your brain? The words you use to describe your current circumstances help form your perceptions of your experiences.

Stress isn't the result of what's occurring in your life. It stems from your *thoughts, feelings* and *perceptions* of what's happening. The words you choose will convey those thoughts and feelings.

How do you describe your life to others? How does your self-talk make you feel?

We are what we believe we are.

There are words we say that feel really good, and there are some that make us cringe just by thinking about them. For example, when you think of the word *peace*, it may produce images of natural beauty, people smiling or a memory of a quiet moment.

If you think about the word *disaster*, there are a whole different set of images and meanings that present themselves. Imagine speaking with a friend or a loved one and describing your day as a disaster. Whether you elaborate or not, images stemming from the concept of a disastrous day have just been reinforced in your brain. By thinking of the word *disaster* repetitively, it will become much easier to create a disaster of a day.

Words have the potential to evoke elaborate images which can elicit strong emotions based on the meaning you've previously assigned to them.

Using negative, insulting or hurtful words not only affects the mood of the person with whom you are speaking, it will also affect you. Choosing to call someone by a demeaning name, making fun of them or treating them poorly has a dual negative effect both on the recipient as well as the speaker. When a person thinks negatively, it is their own nervous system and brain that creates a stress response just by thinking and then saying the words aloud. Negative thoughts can create enough incoherence to permeate every aspect of your being and reduce the optimal communication required between all the systems in your body in order to function and heal optimally.

Conversely, by consciously choosing words that are positive, uplifting and inspiring, you can set a completely different tone that results in a positive environment or circumstance for both the person speaking and the person receiving the words.

Consciously choosing positive words and refraining from speaking negatively towards others is inherently good for you and helps facilitate renewing rather than depleting emotions.

Recording a coherent version of yourself

When you are in a good mood or you feel elevated emotions, it's common to feel like your mind is clearer. Words seem to come easier and you feel empowered when you speak. When you feel coherent, the vibration and energy behind your tone of voice is powerful, balanced and intentional.

Imagine being in a circumstance where you feel sad, angry, anxious or just tired and you're unable to consciously change your vibration and move into a more coherent state. This is extremely common but frustrating for most people because they feel stuck when they can't change their perception of the situation they are in.

Now imagine that when you need encouragement and support, you play a recording of yourself speaking in an elevated and empowered manner, reciting all the uplifting messages you'd want to hear. The recording can be extremely detailed for specific issues or it can focus on eliciting powerful renewing emotions through the use of positive affirmations such as, 'I love you,' 'I am enough,' 'I believe in you' and 'I'm a huge success.'

Here are some helpful tips to get the most out of this exercise:

- Spend as much time as it takes to get into a coherent state. The more sincerity, intention, awareness and energy you use, the more effective this exercise will be. Here are some things you may choose to do to help you attain your desired emotional state: exercise, listen to music, smile, watch a movie, eat mindfully, talk with a friend, do yoga, meditate.

- Create a simple script of words, phrases or sayings that you would like to hear. What motivates you? What do you really want to hear someone say to you? When you are most worried, what can someone say to you that will help? What types of things would your inner, insecure child want to hear?

- Use a recording device on your phone, tablet or computer to record the script you wrote. Be very conscious to enunciate your words well and remember that your tone of voice is just as important as the meaning of the words themselves.

This exercise is beneficial on many levels. First, it is an extremely grounding experience that brings you into the present moment. As you listen to something empowering, you stop ruminating on stressful thoughts. Second, you are receiving incredible messages. Remember, say everything and anything you've ever wanted to hear. Third, and most importantly, it is your own voice. Not only is it your voice, it is your voice when you are *coherent*, when you are *empowered*, when you are *in love*. Even if you listen back to the recording minutes, hours or days later, the words will carry the tone, the energy, the meaning and the memory of the time you were in coherence. You are literally teaching your cells how to be coherent by using a coherent version of yourself.

If you do not have technology to record your script, keep it somewhere safe where you can access it and say it aloud during these moments. Even if you do not feel it at the time, repeat it and yield into the words. Breathe and give yourself the space to repeat the words without judgment. Your cells will hear the words. Allow yourself time to shift your energy. Repeat.

Remember, the more coherent you are, the easier it becomes to recognize when your brain and body feel out of alignment. Engaging in these exercises can become very enjoyable as you awaken your power and ability to support yourself. Have fun with this exercise!

***

TASTE COHERENCE

***

Taste coherence occurs when the taste of any ingestible substance stimulates or increases coherence in any aspect of your being and helps you access renewing emotional states.

***

The taste of food can produce strong chemical and emotional responses that affect the level of coherence throughout your entire body.

Nature does its best to communicate and help you thrive in your environment by providing warning signs and hints as to which foods are beneficial and which should be avoided. There are plants and other types of vegetation that stimulate reactions to their taste which are meant to inform you if they are good or bad for you. Years ago, I went on a fascinating rainforest walk in Brazil where the guide explained how to know which foods were poisonous and which were edible. In the jungle, it is important to understand factors such as colour, location and texture as well as taste and smell.

In nature, many of the foods that are good for you also taste good. It's not usually as simple when it comes to processed, man-made foods. Although packaged food can taste delicious, that does not mean it is good for you. In many cases, it's the exact opposite. Obviously, the ingredients of the food and its nutritional content play a huge role in creating coherence, but even the taste of food can have a huge impact. The taste of some foods can be depleting enough that you avoid them or uplifting enough that you crave them.

It can be challenging when you enjoy the taste of a specific food but it's bad for you or you have a hard time digesting it. Moderation and being in tune with your intention and purpose for eating the specific foods will help you make the best decision in any situation.

There are many healing philosophies, systems and modalities where tastes are used to support the body. Two good examples are Ayurvedic medicine and traditional Eastern-based approaches to healing. According to Ayurvedic medicine, there are various tastes that support different ailments and it's believed that it's important to include some of each in your diet.

Some Eastern-based medicine practitioners recommend eating more bitter-tasting foods for periods of time. They also advise people whether to eat foods that are warming or cooling based on their needs.

Food choices can seem limiting in some situations. It's important to find options that are appealing to your taste buds so that your healing journey is met with increased ease and comfort.

As you go through your coherence journey, pay attention to the tastes that appeal to you and have fun discovering which tastes support you as you experience different emotions.

OLFACTORY COHERENCE

Olfactory coherence results when any smell stimulates or increases coherence in any aspect of your being and helps you access renewing emotional states.

The sense of smell has the capability to both trigger or eliminate a stress response. You can use it to wake up or to help you fall asleep. Specific smells can trigger memories, cause a sneeze or literally result in illness or vomiting.

Using the sense of smell is an effective way to evoke specific emotions.

Some of the more common renewing smells include flowers, fresh air, nature, baked goods, citrus and scented soaps.

Depleting smells include cigarettes, pollution, gas, onions, rotten food and alcohol.

The use of essential oils in vaporizers or sprays is one way to use the sense of smell to elicit different moods and create more coherence. The sense of smell is unique to each person. While a scent may be invigorating and renewing for one person, the same scent may be offensive and depleting for another. By exploring different smells, you can become aware of which oils evoke specific emotional states in you.

Exploration of scents. Are there scents that will enhance the start of your day or make your shower more enjoyable? What smells would motivate you during your drive to work or at your office? Are there rooms in your home where you can utilize essential oils? Are there specific spices that you would like to cook with?

Explore and discover the benefits for your being so you can use the sense of smell to increase coherence in as many aspects of your life as you can.

Using essential oils to create different emotional states

Here's a list of 10 popular essential oils and the health benefits associated with them:

- Peppermint: to boost energy and aid digestion,

- Lavender: to relieve stress,

- Sandalwood: to calm nerves and help with focus,

- Bergamot: to reduce stress and improve skin conditions like eczema,

- Rose: to improve mood and reduce anxiety,

- Chamomile: to improve mood and relaxation,

- Ylang-ylang: to treat headaches, nausea and skin conditions,

- Tea tree: to fight infections and boost immunity,

- Jasmine: to help with depression, childbirth and libido,

- Lemon: to aid digestion, mood, headaches and more.
  (https://www.healthline.com/nutrition/what-are-essential-oils#types)

Chapter 16

DIGESTIVE COHERENCE

_____

Digestive coherence is the optimal process that occurs as the body breaks down food into the most effective and efficient building blocks used to produce fuel and energy for the body.

_____

Science has discovered that humans actually have three brains: the one in your head, the heart brain and the gut brain. The gut brain is an intricate network of neural tissue that sends an enormous amount of information from the digestive system directly to the brain. This is one way of understanding your gut instinct and how it connects to a sense of intuition because the digestive system is constantly communicating with both your heart and brain.

Some people achieve digestive coherence by eating a basic diet, while for others, it can be incredibly complicated to find foods that satisfy their nutritional needs and sensitivities. One quick search of the internet will demonstrate how many different options you have. It can be overwhelming.

There are high-protein and low-fat diets. There are ketogenic, paleo, macrobiotic, vegan and organic approaches. You can follow the Medical Medium. You can sign up for Jenny Craig, Weight Watchers or you can simply count your calories. You can eat throughout the day or intermittently fast. Many people choose to be vegetarians while others eat meat. The options seem endless.

One of the most powerful ways to increase or decrease coherence in your body is through your diet. From the moment you place food in your mouth (or even sooner if you smell the food), your body begins to secrete chemical messengers known as enzymes that help your body break down and digest the food. The goal of your digestive system is to ensure that the nutrients provided can be absorbed, assimilated and processed for energy on a cellular level. During optimal digestion, your body breaks down and utilizes all foods effectively and efficiently in order to reap the maximum benefits.

There are many factors that go into determining whether a food is coherent with your body, including food sensitivities, allergies, fluctuating hormone levels, stress level and how much processing the food went through.

It's important to remember that when your body, mind and spirit are misaligned and your emotions are out of sorts, it is much more difficult to digest foods effectively. When your body is in coherence and you experience elevated emotions, it tends to be easier to digest food.

Increased energy, a boosted immune response, effective healing and elevated emotions are just some of the benefits of a coherent digestive system. Creating a plan to explore your diet will help you determine the best foods for you.

Explore your diet

Step 1. Written exercise

To start this process, track everything you eat for three to five days. Using our tracking sheet or in your journal, record how you feel before, during and 30 minutes after the meal. Make sure to note any symptoms in your body, your energy level as well as your mood.

If your intention is to create a plan that satisfies your nutritional goals, it is important to enjoy the food. Otherwise, your commitment won't last. I suggest as you're tracking the food you eat, you rate how much you enjoyed specific foods. It will help you decide what to eliminate and what to keep in your diet. Remember that while a certain food may be deemed 'healthy' or as a 'superfood', if you have a sensitivity to it, it will not be a superfood for you.

Helpful questions to ask yourself:

- Were you bloated? Did your abdomen feel distended?

- Did you like the taste?

- Was it easy to make? How long did it take?

- What mood were you in immediately after? Thirty minutes after?

- Were you energized, relaxed, anxious?

- Would you make this a regular meal?

- How did this meal affect your elimination?

Step 2. Elimination diet

The purpose of an elimination diet is to rule out any food sensitivities or intolerances. After you've completed the first week and reviewed your remarks you will know which foods are coherent or incoherent with your body. If you take the time to rate each meal you can keep a list of meals you want to repeat. Now it's time to go through step 1 again by creating new meals for the week and going through the same process.

Step 3. Eight-five-three

After you go through steps 1 and 2 (as many times as you'd like), you will have many options and will be ready to create a diet with various suitable options for meals, snacks and beverages. For some people, committing to a meal plan seems rigid. While for others, it is freeing to have a system to follow.

If following a specific plan does not resonate with you, I suggest creating lists that you can refer to when you're looking for meal options. The lists can be divided into different categories, such as meal options and snacks, as well as groups identifying foods that can help you relax, increase energy or attain specific moods when necessary.

If you are looking to create a customized system you can follow, I have found that following an 8-5-3 system reduces stress and can set you up for success.

An 8-5-3 meal plan consists of eight dinners, five lunches and three breakfasts. Typically, this system provides you with more options than your current diet. The great thing about implementing this is that it is completely flexible and adaptable. If you follow it the majority of the time, you will ensure that you are eating foods that help you accomplish your health goals. You can change it and make substitutions at any time. I suggest that you assess your meals every three months or so and change as much or as little as you would like. Some people make very few changes to their 8-5-3 system over an entire year while others enjoy changing at least two to three meals every time they assess the plan.

Creating a coherent eating plan

For your plan to truly be coherent with your life, it has to accomplish more than just providing you the proper nutrition. It's important to consider other criteria when it comes to your diet, such as viability, budget and convenience, as these factors may be creating incoherence and stress in your life. I have spoken to many patients who have had challenges committing to their plan due to the cost. Buying food that is organic or unprocessed can be prohibitive. I recommend creating a budget and pricing out all the ingredients to the meals you choose. This will also address the issue of where to buy the ingredients. You will definitely reduce any tension you have around your diet by creating a menu that includes food you can afford and know where to purchase.

It is also important to consider how much time, effort and skill is needed. Many people feel intimidated when facing the daunting task of making healthy food for themselves. It is helpful to learn how to prepare each meal and budget the time in your schedule.

Once you are proficient at preparing the meals, the only thing left to do is enjoy eating them!

Chapter 17

THE SIXTH SENSE – INTUITION

Each of us has an inner voice that is meant to guide us. The reality, though, is that it's usually drowned by our analytical mind.

You know the voice I'm talking about. It's the one that tells you right from wrong, good from bad and always has your best interest at heart. It's that gut instinct you get, the feeling some people call 'having a hunch.'

There are some people who easily pick up on energy and receive strong energy messages. These people are often referred to as 'intuitives' or 'empaths.'

_____

Intuitive empaths are highly sensitive people that can sense subtle energies, emotions and physical symptoms from others and absorb that energy into their own bodies. It is often difficult for empaths to distinguish someone else's discomfort from their own. (www.drjudithorloff.com)

_____

Intuition can be the force that guides you toward a particular person in the room. It can also be the nagging apprehension you feel when you are uncertain about an upcoming decision or the unquestionable deep knowing that you are on the right track.

Although it may not always make sense or seem logical, it's important to listen to that voice and be aware of what your intuition is telling you even if it seems like the last thing you want to do. You will make better decisions in your life when you pay attention to your inner voice.

Achieving Zen during fight or flight

———————————

Fight-or-flight Zen. The ability of the average person, who is stuck in a stress response (experiences constant fight or flight), to gain control over their emotional state by listening to their coherent *intuitive voice.*

———————————

Over the course of many years, expressing and releasing my emotions through tears was common. It was common for me to create a cathartic experience to reset my emotional state. Eventually I developed a comfort level within the panic and became aware of my calm inner voice. I essentially developed the ability to talk myself through intense emotional situations. I found the ability to access a calming, coherent internal voice in the midst of a stressful event or even a panic attack.

The voice would say things like, 'While I'm letting this out, should I start to make lunch?' I'd literally be in the middle of breaking down and listening to my inner voice saying, 'This is good. It feels nice to cry. I'm feeling sorry for myself right now but if I don't get going, I'll be late and won't have time to get my work done.'

In the midst of overreacting or when I couldn't attribute the intense anxiety I was feeling to anything, I found the voice very practical and rational. It would encourage me to go take a shower, meditate, smile, call someone or do whatever I needed to do in that moment to increase my coherence.

The better I got at regulating my emotional responses through breathwork, the easier it became to listen to my inner calming voice.

The message and tone of the voice is calm and often at odds with the intensity of the situation. When I stop and listen, it helps me return to the present moment and gain clarity. This always reduces the intensity and duration of the stressful episode.

Chapter 18

CAREER AND FINANCIAL COHERENCE

CAREER COHERENCE

Career coherence occurs when the job or career you choose inspires you, gives you purpose, easily funds your lifestyle and facilitates renewal of your emotional system.

Whether you are just starting your career or you have decided to reassess your goals, it's important for you to be very clear on what type of job or career you would like to have.

Even if you do not currently have your dream job, if you are open to new ideas, then it's still possible. When considering all of your choices, I suggest following a few fundamental principles. The first principle is to set an intention to do something that you enjoy every day. The second principle is to do something that will inspire you and give you purpose. Lastly, your ideal career or job should easily fund the lifestyle you have chosen to live. For your career to be coherent with the rest of your life, it is extremely important to enjoy what you do, recognize its value and earn enough money from it.

Some people can exist on a relatively small amount of money, while others choose to live luxuriously. Getting clear on the funds necessary for your lifestyle is an eye-opening and extremely valuable exercise.

In addition to understanding the affordability of the lifestyle you've chosen, there are other questions that will help ensure you are making the right choices:

1. If you've decided to make a change: How did you originally choose? Money? Joy? Path of least resistance?

2. What other considerations were there? Did you follow the crowd? Did you cave in to pressure? Did a family member or friend inspire you? Do you want to follow in someone's footsteps? Can you talk with them?

3. Are you working but still searching? Do you like to change jobs every few years?

4. If you're just starting out, what would you enjoy doing every day? What are you good at? What makes you smile and excites you to get out of bed in the morning?

5. Do you want the security of a job or is it your goal to own a business?

6. What hours do you want to work?

7. What are you physically capable of?

8. How does the career you chose affect your health?

9. What environments do you enjoy spending time in? Where are you productive?

10. Do you want to work with a team or on your own?

Creating and implementing an action plan after answering all of the relevant questions will give you the best chance of manifesting your desired career and creating a balanced life.

As you begin to explore opportunities, it is very helpful to identify and practice the specific emotions you want to feel while doing your dream job. The more familiar the emotion feels, the easier it becomes to feel the emotion.

FINANCIAL COHERENCE

_____

Financial coherence occurs when your job / career or your investments result in enough wealth to create and manifest your financial desires. The financial stress you've experienced in the past can be released by developing an understanding and a belief that you will always have enough. Ultimately, *financial coherence* leads to financial freedom.

_____

One of the most common and overwhelming stressors people deal with in their lives is financial stress. Your belief systems start to develop early and are affected by the circumstances you've gone through. You may have seen the struggles your parents went through or perhaps you have developed fear based on perceived failures or other types of challenges. Your journey may have required sacrificing and prioritizing, or perhaps your choices simply did not produce the results you were expecting. Many people feel like they are fighting an uphill battle because their subconscious beliefs are working against them. Do you have a core belief that you will always have enough? Once you understand what *enough* means to you, it's much easier to install or reinforce that concept.

Dream life exercise

It can be extremely eye opening to gain clarity and understand how much your dream life will actually cost. Some people conclude that they do not need nearly as much money to live their dream life as they thought, while for others, it can be a harsh dose of reality.

Typically, many people want to earn millions of dollars per year while having their dream job. Who wouldn't want that, right?

What if you calculated that to live your dream life, it would cost $450,000/year? What if your dream life only cost $100,000/year? I'm not suggesting that you don't aim high. I'm suggesting that after you have determined exactly what it will cost to live your dream life, there is no need to unnecessarily burden yourself with the pressure of needing more success. Hopefully, designing and creating your dream life is enough.

Here are some questions and topics to consider while calculating the expenses of your dream life:

- basic costs of living: accommodation, cars, utilities, taxes, groceries / food;

- health expense, insurance;

- hobbies: what do you enjoy doing?

- vacations: how often and how many, which destinations?

- investments;

- presents, charities;

- include anything you desire and don't be conservative – this is your dream.

Once you have created a detailed plan and are aware of how much your dream life will cost, you can make a plan to attain it. I suggest that you review it every few months and revise it according to your current circumstances and goals.

Chapter 19

SOCIAL COHERENCE AND COHERENT COMMUNICATION

Coherent communication, as defined by The HeartMath Institute, is the process of aligning energetically, whether two people or many, in order for there to be a high value placed on listening and making sure the speaker feels heard. The goal of *coherent communication* processes is to transcend the 'noise' of regular human communication by listening to feelings as well as words, and for all participants to commit to staying as mentally and emotionally coherent as possible during the communications.

Coherent communication, therefore, is a result of any words, gestures, interactions or body language that stimulate or increase coherence in any aspect of your being and helps access renewing emotional states.

Social coherence is the result of the harmony or resonance between human beings. Coherence is created at a cellular level when the electromagnetic fields of different people interact. An attraction or affinity towards each other is formed.

One of the most fundamental aspects of life is that we are social beings. We have families and create communities to serve many purposes. We look outwards for support, love, companionship and conversation. Communication between human beings can take many forms including physical touch, spoken word, gestures, body language as well as less understood methods such as our electromagnetic fields.

We each have an electromagnetic field that radiates outwards from our body that can give us feedback as to whether we are in or out of coherence with someone else.

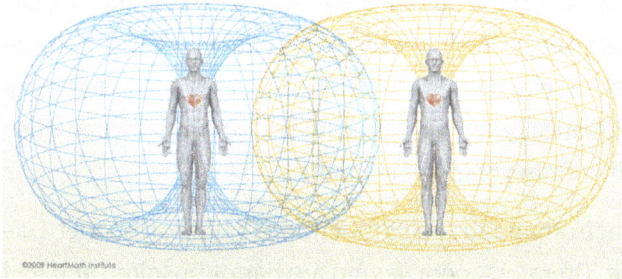

Image courtesy of the HeartMath® Institute – www.heartmath.org

When you click with someone, you can literally *feel it*. Sometimes you can feel a connection right away during an introductory handshake. Other times you may not have a sense of your connection until you've spoken or spent significant time together. Some conversations flow with ease while on other occasions, someone may irritate or annoy you with their voice alone.

Nonverbal communication is extremely important. I'm sure you've had an experience where you received a hug from a friend and realized it was exactly what you needed.

You can *feel* a look or even a twinkle in an eye. Humans feel emotion due to subtle gestures made by those around them.

A good way to illustrate *social coherence* is to think about a situation when you felt really happy or uplifted as soon as a specific person entered the room and you instantly wanted to talk with them. Contrast that with another occasion when you saw someone and felt an internal contraction leading to a perception of negative energy. You most likely wanted to avoid that person or go into another room.

What is the difference? Your cells can literally be in coherence with one person and not with the other. Ideally, you would always want to be in coherence with those around you. However, we all spend time with people whose vibration either adds or detracts from our level of coherence.

When you are truly conscious in your interactions, you can gain a great deal of clarity about who depletes and who renews you. You can then use that understanding to your advantage. When you make the commitment to surround yourself with people who renew you, it conserves your vital energy and increases your joy for life. It is also accurate to say that your energy is drastically less depleted when you avoid spending time with people with whom you don't resonate.

Our electromagnetic fields function as a type of magnet. Like generally attracts like. Therefore, people who are happy, inspired and joyful tend to attract those types of people into their lives.

When you start to realize how precious your time and energy are, you will protect both. Spending time with people who renew you rather than deplete you makes a huge impact on your energy level, mood and perception of your day.

Surrounding yourself with people who renew you results in that extra boost you may need as motivation to go to the gym or the energy you need to cook dinner when you get home. It's the difference between making the effort to call an old friend or continuing to put it off. Will you flop into bed and crash, or be alert enough to read your book before bed?

When you feel depleted around specific people and their vibe or energy doesn't resonate with you, it's not their fault. There doesn't have to be judgment and it's okay if you don't feel your best around them. It's a positive outcome to be able to discern who is healthy for you and who you may choose to stay away from as you maintain your level of coherence.

Once you commit to the process of elevating your coherence level, you will see powerful shifts in the amount of *social coherence* you experience. As I mentioned above, the more coherent you are, the more you attract similarly coherent people into your life. Conversely, when you're coherent, if people whom you no longer feel a resonance with enter your life, you are able to approach them with a sense of grace and ease. You are able to make choices that suit you in respectful ways. You can send love to others even if you do not resonate with them because you know that it's simply a different frequency.

Knowing how to use *social coherence* for growth

Creating *social coherence* consciously can be an effective neurological interrupt. In other words, once you understand how other people's energy affects you and how your energy affects them, you can start to use *social coherence* to grow in times of need. When it is hard for you to evoke a positive emotion in yourself or change your physiological state, you can elevate your own emotion by eliciting a strong emotional response in someone. For example, if you want to improve your own mood, make an effort to do something for someone else such as buying a coffee for the person behind you in line. The gratitude they feel will help create the same emotion in you. That is the power of *social coherence*! When you connect with others, your physiology will change. Doing something, such as a random act of kindness, to make other people happy is just as impactful for you as it is for the other person.

Selfishly altruistic

Performing authentic acts of loving kindness has a direct positive effect on your own health. By creating genuine feelings of care, love, generosity or appreciation, your brain will trigger the release of hormones and happy chemicals (see Appendix), which facilitate healing and leave you feeling good.

When circumstances arise that leave you feeling unable to lift your mood or feel positive, it can be helpful to say or do something positive for someone else. When you tell someone they are beautiful, smart or loved, you also feel equally as good. If you engage in an act that improves someone else's day, you will benefit from a positive shift.

Humor me here. I want to strongly encourage you to do something seemingly altruistic and loving for someone, but I want you to do it for yourself. Be a little selfish – just to be playful with this concept. Engage in as many loving gestures as you can but consciously do them for your own benefit and let others enjoy the outcome.

Control your mind space

Another habit many people have is letting themselves get depleted by the words or actions of people they barely know or spend time with. I spent many years focused on the opinions of those around me. Whether it was close friends or strangers, I allowed other people to impact the way I felt about myself.

As you gain emotional control and operate from a perspective of renewal, it becomes easier to identify people who take up too much space in your mind. Every time you increase your coherence in any aspect of your life, you gain the ability to take back a little more control of your thoughts and actions.

The older I get, the more this concept resonates with me. I would like to emphasize again, though, that your sense of self-worth has nothing to do with other people. They are not to blame. This is about you.

You experience many scenarios in your life for the specific purpose of learning and growth. When you become a conscious observer of yourself, you become more aware of how you focus your energy, attention and thoughts. Rather than placing blame on people or events in your external world, you can regain your self-worth and self-esteem by looking within, healing your wounds, connecting with your lessons and making empowered choices.

It is always up to you to decide where you place your thoughts and focus your energy. As you begin your journey through the *Coherence Revolution*, you may feel compelled to connect with people who have *not* been coherent with you in the past. It's important to discern the value and investment in these relationships. Remember, you are in control of *you*. You have the choice. As your journey continues, you will recognize and develop your ability to attract people, scenarios and experiences which are in coherence with the life you wish to lead.

Chapter 20

NATURAL COHERENCE

The goal of life is to make your heartbeat match the beat of the universe,
to match your nature with nature.
— Joseph Campbell

Natural coherence occurs when any aspect of the natural world stimulates or helps facilitate more coherence in any aspect of your being and helps access renewing emotional states.

We all have experiences in life that seem to flow perfectly and feel right. These are the times when you have a sense of clarity about your life and the world seems to make sense. During these times there are actually significant changes occurring in your brain.

Each specific brain wave frequency can induce a wide variety of physiological states and moods ranging from stressed out and frustrated to creative, happy, calm and peaceful.

Our planet is full of natural elements that can be used to create coherence and help your brain shift from depleting, stressful brain wave patterns into more renewing and healthy ones.

There is a fundamental interconnectedness between humans and the Earth that impacts all of us. There are also many different vibrational frequencies that permeate our atmosphere, interact with our brain and nervous systems, and help us achieve renewed emotional states. The better you understand the interaction between yourself and the planet, the more effectively you can use it to your advantage throughout your life.

Spending time in natural environments such as our rivers, forests and mountains will facilitate a higher volume of brainwaves in the high alpha and theta frequency range. That is why you feel more inspired, relaxed and healthy when you spend a day at the beach, enjoy a hike in the mountains or go for a walk in the woods.

Urban environments generally operate and vibrate in the more stressful frequency ranges such as high beta waves. There is a big difference between the way your brain functions and adapts to stress when you take a walk through a park versus down Main Street. A depleting response is created when you spend time in stressful environments such as streets filled with stoplights, pollution, cars, cement, buildings and visual chaos.

We all experience environments that stimulate more stressful high beta brain waves. They're hard to completely avoid. Typically, I'm talking about an office environment, the shopping mall, becoming stuck in traffic or walking around downtown in the city.

The more aware you are of your surroundings and the types of environments you spend time in, the more consciously you can use your surroundings to adapt to any stressful circumstance that arises.

One of my greatest passions in life is spending time exploring everything nature has to offer. Whether it's a short walk in the forest, a camping trip, scuba diving, waterfall hunting or skiing in the mountains, once you find what resonates with you, natural coherence is a powerful tool you always have at your disposal.

Water has always been an environment I've thrived in. My parents taught me to swim at a young age, and I've always enjoyed and felt comfortable in the water. There is a feeling of peace that comes over me when I'm immersed. I feel free. From swimming and boating to scuba diving and cliff jumping, I've spent a lot of time and have experienced many adventures in the water.

Some of the most peaceful and joyful moments of my life are directly related to water. One of my best memories from childhood was when I entered and won the senior shift swim marathon as a member of the junior shift. It was my claim to fame at summer camp for many years because as a junior shift camper, I was only 11 years old. I remember being so proud of myself for beating all the older kids!

It came as no surprise to me that when I finally learned how to scuba dive in my early thirties, it quickly became one of my biggest passions. There is nowhere I feel more calm or mindful.

I do my best to spend as much time in the water as possible.

I have always found mountains to have a spiritual aura. They have a majestic quality and mystery about them. Science has shown that mountains generally vibrate in the theta frequency range, which is why it is so calming to sit on top of a mountain and look at the surrounding landscape.

I have always had a craving to spend as much time as I can in the mountains and there have been several times in my life that I came close to moving to Western Canada. Although that never happened, my passion for spending time in the mountains is just as strong as it's ever been. I will participate in just about any activity as long as it's in the mountains: skiing, hiking, biking, rappelling, climbing, canyoning and photography.

My first ski trip was in 1986 when I went to Banff, Canada, with some friends. I was only 15 years old. Since then I have experienced many adventures; and I've explored mountains in Whistler, New Zealand, Australia, Austria, Quebec, Fernie BC, the Grand Tetons, Utah, Jasper, Jackson Hole, Zion National Park, Bryce Canyon and Revelstoke, just to name a few.

The memories of the time I've spent in the mountains are very vivid and are good examples of how past experiences can elicit an emotion. I frequently use those trips as part of my visualizations while doing HeartMath. It is a lot of fun to relive each of my trips and experience some of those emotions again.

There are many cultures which encourage people to respectfully interact with the planet and discover, through investigation, which elements and natural resources are best utilized for one's health and balance. Elements such as water, fire, air, earth and ether are just a few. I encourage you to spend some time in nature to discover where you feel grounded, invigorated, connected and at ease. These are valuable tools for your personal coherence journey.

Chapter 21

GLOBAL COHERENCE

Global coherence is the most optimal state of our planet as it relates to human existence and its place within the galaxy and the entire universe.

The relationship between humans and the planet is meant to be a reciprocal relationship. Although mankind has begun an effort to help the planet heal and change our destructive path, we haven't lived up to our end of the bargain quite yet.

Humans, animals, plants, organisms and all living things are meant to be in coherence with each other. There is a growing body of research in the fields of quantum science, neurophysiology, psychology and mathematics that is essentially proving just that.

At times, it may not seem that events around the globe are connected, but the higher the vantage point you view humanity from, the clearer the organized chaos becomes.

The earth's electromagnetic field is composed of many different frequencies, and we are only beginning to understand the relevant impact of each of them.

The HeartMath Institute has been pioneering research and seeking new methods to consciously improve *global coherence* of Earth's vibrational frequencies. They call it *The Global Coherence Initiative*. The purpose is to unite people in heart-focused love and intention to facilitate the shift in *global* consciousness from instability and discord to compassionate care, cooperation and increasing peace.

They're asking two key questions: can we cause and create more coherence in the Earth's electromagnetic field? Can we heal the planet by creating more coherence in the field?

It is extremely powerful and personally healing to spend time connecting with thousands of other people with the joint intention of healing our planet.

Section 4

LIVING A COHERENT LIFE

Chapter 22

KEY CONCEPTS FOR LIVING A COHERENT LIFE

Coherence does not mean relaxation, but it can be very relaxing.

One common assumption is that coherence is merely a state of relaxation. It is true that to be truly relaxed, you must be in coherence. However, if you are coherent, you are not necessarily relaxed. Being coherent is being in a state of rhythm and flow, whether the emotion is excited, happy, peaceful, calm or content.

When you are in coherence, your emotional state is pure, and it allows you to utilize and conserve your energy appropriately and efficiently. The circumstance will dictate whether the result will be increased energy or a more relaxed state.

You may find yourself in a situation where you are experiencing a lot of stress and your mind is racing. The intention behind getting coherent, in this case, is to achieve a state of relaxation, reduce your heart rate and slow down the thought process.

Other circumstances can be quite different. Imagine being at home feeling lonely, stressed and anxious, when a friend texts you to meet them in an hour for dinner with a bunch of people. The most effective way to ensure it is a positive experience and a renewing situation would be to increase your coherence level and change your emotional state. Rather than trying to relax or calm your mind, the intention behind creating coherence in this scenario would be to energize your body. You can choose the renewing emotions that are congruent with the uplifting environment you would be anticipating when you meet your friends for dinner.

What is incoherence and how does it affect your life?

If we know what coherence is, then don't we also know what incoherence is? Well, yes and no. If you are not coherent, then yes, to some degree, you are incoherent.

What does that mean practically? We've all experienced it. At its basic level, if a system is incoherent, it is not in balance. When referring to the human body, if it's not in a state of flow or balance, it can be said to be in a state of dis-ease.

In exactly the same way that coherence affects all of our senses, tissues, cells and emotions, so does incoherence. If your eyes are not functioning well and cannot interpret images in a coherent manner, then you may need glasses. If sound waves aren't interpreted coherently, you may not hear what someone is trying to communicate. If your brain does not interpret your current situation as coherent, you will most likely experience a stress response.

In general, when your cells do not receive coherent signals from the brain, they will not function properly or be able to replicate perfectly. It is said that every seven years, you are a new you. Although different tissues in your body replicate at different rates, seven years from now, there will not be a single cell left in your body that exists today. If this process carried on and every one of your cells, in every tissue, replicated perfectly, you would live forever.

As humans, we all age at different rates based upon our genetic code and our level of health. When incoherent patterns infiltrate every aspect of your life, your cells will not replicate or function perfectly any longer. This is called a state of dis-ease. Essentially, you don't work as well, and it requires a greater amount of energy to keep your body functioning. Your body can only be out of balance, operating in a dysfunctional way, for so long before dis-ease in specific systems becomes diagnosed as a health condition and an actual disease.

Just let it go

'Cheer up, calm down, take it easy, be happy, don't worry. Just do it!' Easy, right?

How about, 'Get over it, let it go, be in the moment, be mindful, be grateful, get your mind off it, don't sweat the small stuff, life is too short'?

Feel better now? Maybe, but possibly not.

Letting go seems so simple, yet it can be one of the hardest things you'll ever have to do.

If you pay attention, you'll realize how often someone says one of those statements to you or you say them to yourself when you are trying to reduce your stress and solve your problems.

Love does heal. Getting your mind off it will help. Being mindful and staying in the moment does reduce anxiety. Life is too short. If all of those things are true, why is it so hard to actually do?

It comes down to effort. Believe it or not, it is much easier to allow yourself to feel stressed than to do something about it. It is easier to complain than to heal. It is easier to blame than to take responsibility.

A large part of why people don't simply *let go* is very practical. You have to learn *how* to let go, which can be a process that requires consistent practice and focus. Some people have a hard time finding methods that work for them, some get frustrated by techniques they don't quite grasp and others are not consistent enough to see the results.

The other reason it can be challenging to just *let go* is because when you are in the middle of a stress response, you either want to fight, flee or completely freeze on the spot. That's why the response is called *fight or flight (or freeze)*. Most people are unable to come up with a plan of action or motivation to do anything when they're experiencing panic. It becomes very hard to process information accurately and efficiently when the mind ruminates and races. The result is usually an incoherent, irrational response.

If you have ever suffered with anxiety or panic, you will have had occasions where you were sitting at home feeling anxious or depressed and felt helpless. In those situations, it can take a herculean effort to do even the simplest of self-care techniques. Yet if you took just 30 seconds and smiled in front of a mirror, your physiology would begin to change instantly and your perception of the entire episode could change.

The energy barrier feels insurmountable but if you were just able to turn on your favorite music and force yourself to dance, listen to some personal affirmations or do any number of things you've identified as part of this course, you can literally change your entire circumstance.

The sooner you can break the stress response and create some coherence, the sooner you can make some good decisions and think from a different state of mind and a much healthier place.

It's the times you choose to surrender that bring healing. Forgiving yourself and others doesn't make you weak; it sets you free. Once you spend time increasing coherence, it is much easier to let go of the battles that can leave you *bitter* so you can go after your *better*.

Release yourself from carrying the pain of the past because a bad chapter does not mean an unhappy life. Stay in the present, gain coherence and create your peace.

Creating coherence in every aspect of your life results in your optimal timeline

My healing journey has spanned several decades. Over the last several years concepts from a variety of books and courses have suddenly come together to make sense like never before. It's been like fitting in the last few pieces of a puzzle to finally see the whole picture.

Traditional science tells us that life consists of a finite linear timeline. If you're like most people, you have an intention to achieve specific goals and create the best life you possibly can.

In a typical scenario, you might have a specific financial or career goal that motivates you to read some books, learn the right skills and find the best teachers. In other words, you try to do everything right. Does that mean you will achieve the goal? No, not necessarily, but there are some really good signs you're heading in the right direction.

If you're an overachiever or consider yourself a type-A personality, success is not determined by what you're doing for each particular project or goal. You know you will commit to getting your goal accomplished. You know you will create a list of things to do. And you know you will stick with your timeline and do what is necessary to accomplish the goal. It's not about whether you are doing enough.

Your success will depend on your mindset, the type of energy you have and the emotional state you are in while trying to accomplish your goal. Ultimately, long-term success will depend on whether you are depleted or renewed.

You cannot achieve your optimal outcome and live your *dream life* while one aspect of yourself is incoherent. For example, it is extremely challenging to create the inspiration necessary to grow your business if you're going through a divorce or experiencing health issues. How can you be innovative at work if you're exhausted from a conversation with your boss? When you're not eating well and your blood sugar levels are low, it's hard to make decisions or evoke a loving feeling towards another.

Incoherence in one area of your life decreases your ability to achieve coherence in all other areas.

Ultimately, it is the most coherent version of yourself that will create your dream life. Quantum scientists believe that at any given moment, there are an infinite number of timelines in our universe. It is theorized that each of the timelines are occurring in the quantum universe at the exact same time and you become aware of the one that matches your vibrational resonance. In other words, your reality will be the one you are in coherence with. If each timeline has the possibility of creating a different future, then your dream life would be the result of the one in which you are the most coherent in every possible way.

Every time you raise your vibration and gain more coherence, you are accessing the potential in the quantum field that is in the most optimal coherence with your dreams and intentions.

In Gregg Braden's book, *Fractal Time,* he talks about the likelihood for something to occur if the proper conditions are present. To clarify, just because the conditions are right for something to occur doesn't mean it will. It may be sunny and beautiful, but it doesn't mean you will choose to go outside, let alone go to the beach.

You may feel ready for love, money or friendship; but even if the conditions are perfect, you will still have to do what's necessary to make it happen.

Let's say an *opportunity* arises at work for you to advance your career. You may not even be aware of the opportunity yet. In this example, let's assume you wake up each day with a positive attitude and a passion for life. You make a conscious, sincere effort to maximize coherence in all aspects of your life, which also means you have created conditions in your life that are in coherence with the *opportunity*. It could be a promotion, it could be a business idea or it could be a conversation leading to an interview. The *'opportunity'* is the condition in life that is present, and because you have created coherence in all aspects of your life, you matched the coherent frequency of the positive opportunity.

In this way, you have significantly increased the chances of consciously creating the outcome you want.

The opposite is also true. In this scenario, let's assume the same positive opportunity presents itself, except in this case, you have become stressed out, tired and fearful; you're not loving towards yourself or others. Even though the conditions for the opportunity are the same at work, the outcome will not be the same because you are not doing or feeling the same things. Your thoughts and emotional state are not in coherence. This will affect your health, your relationships at work, your attitude and your perception of the environment you're working in.

You can only perceive a situation that has a vibration that is equal to the vibration or level of coherence you are exhibiting. Being less coherent will undoubtedly lead to a different outcome. In fact, most likely, you would never have perceived there was a positive opportunity.

The overwhelming response

As you improve at consciously creating more coherence in your life, you will have the ability to choose the intensity of the emotional response you're practicing. Learning how to subtly change and elevate your mood is very valuable, but to effectively change hardwired programs and significantly alter your response to stressful situations, the emotional response you practice and respond with must be bigger and more powerful than the incoherent pattern or habit that is already there.

Imagine for a moment that you find yourself at home feeling anxious, depressed and completely out of control. Now imagine that your doorbell rings and someone is at the door delivering a package that you needed and you have to sign for. Tough situation, right?

In most cases, things happen pretty quickly and you wouldn't think about it very much. You would immediately switch into a new mode. You would wipe off your tears, pull yourself together, give a quick look in the mirror and answer the door with a big smile on your face. The person would smile back, hand you the package and you would sign for it while exchanging pleasantries.

For a moment, you would be transformed. You wouldn't feel like crying or being depressed. You would not be out of control. You would be in the moment. And I'm betting that it would feel pretty good.

In that scenario, I'm sure a part of you wanted to get rid of whoever it was and close the door so you could literally break down and cry again. *A part of you wanted that very badly.* There was also a part of you that wanted the interaction to last longer because you felt more yourself in that moment than perhaps any other time in recent memory.

In a general sense, worrying about the future results in anxious thoughts and feelings while thinking about stressful past events tends to lead to more depressive thoughts and feelings. The only time that both are absent is in the present moment.

Let's take a look at what happened in the previous example.

Before the doorbell, most likely, you were stuck in a depleting pattern of switching from scary future thoughts to depressing memories. When patterns are hardwired, it doesn't take a lot to trigger the production of your powerful stress hormones. It can get easier and easier to fire up your fight-or-flight response due to the fact you've probably been practicing it for many years. Unfortunately, creating anxiety in your body can become your natural set point.

So what happened when the doorbell rang?

There was a *neurological interrupt* that shocked you back to the present moment. The only thing you had to focus on in that moment was how to make yourself look and sound presentable very quickly.

To answer the door in a calm, socially acceptable way, your response had to be intense, focused and delivered with a lot of intention behind it. If you didn't produce a strong enough positive emotional response, then you would have answered the door in the exact same state as when it rang, crying and anxious.

This may be very specific and even exaggerated, but it is a good example of what is possible. You can change your mood in an instant. It's possible to get rid of anxiety or even depression in a split second if the response is great enough. And if you practice this over and over, you will change your set point, and your depleting automatic responses will diminish.

Throughout all the years of seeking help I found it very unhelpful that so many therapists told me that it would take years to get rid of anxiety. They added to my negative self-talk! It doesn't have to be this way. It can literally take seconds. Conceptually, this is easy stuff, yet it takes a strong commitment to yourself to change.

Create coherence and figure everything else out later

It's reasonable to say that when you are anxious, stressed or generally unwell, it is not the best time to make important decisions or be relied upon. Unfortunately, that's exactly what most people have to do on a daily basis. Whether it's a relationship that needs mending, tasks that need to be done, chores to be accomplished, disasters to avoid or catastrophes to be dealt with, most people are not in their optimal state, in any given moment, to function the way they hoped they would.

So many people constantly feel disappointed with themselves.

You know when you could have done better but haven't because you're not thinking or behaving as your best self. You always know, deep down. You can change the outcomes in your life when you focus on creating coherence before you expect to heal, feel better or move on. Create coherence before you expect yourself to let go. When your mind is confused or overwhelmed and you can't think straight, it's *not* time to make a decision.

When your level of coherence is impacted by a situation, a place, an object or an interaction with a person, it's your choice how you respond. You can spend time and energy trying to figure out what happened and why. You can try and determine who is right and who is wrong. You can make sure the person knows why you feel the way you do.

I suggest the first thing you do is create more coherence in your body, elevate your mood and raise your vibration. In those moments, it's not about being right, proving your point or getting what you want. You are certainly allowed to do all of those things, but none of them will change your situation for the better.

When you are in a stressful or depleting circumstance, it may appear that you have no choice. You may feel that you have done nothing to create the situation you find yourself in. You may be frustrated.

In these negative types of mindset, it is especially important to be able to think about the situation clearly. These are the times to listen to your intuitive inner voice.

By focusing on creating more coherence in the moment, you are preparing yourself to handle the circumstance in the most optimal way, whatever way it goes. Yes, this could feel like you're ignoring the problem temporarily. Yes, that's true. Yes, you will not pay attention to what could have happened. Yes, if there is a person involved, you may not receive what you were seeking.

The most loving thing you can do for yourself in these situations is to focus on getting into a coherent state. If that means dancing all alone in your bedroom, taking a walk in nature, getting in a cold shower, watching a comedy, painting, meditating, breathing, writing, singing, holding hands or hugging a loved one, do whatever it takes.

The circumstance will seem much less complicated after you've become coherent. Many times the issue you thought you had really wasn't as bad as you feared or it resolved itself altogether. In fact, you may not even be able to remember why it was so upsetting. But if the problem does still exist, it will be less overwhelming and you will be able to find a heart-centered response to whatever is going on.

Most of us just want to be heard, understood, proved right or validated. I know I do. But if you're honest with yourself, that's not usually the core issue. When you are comfortable and in coherence with all of your decisions, it doesn't matter what others think or feel about you. This is not meant in a rude or self-centered manner. It's not ego. It's awareness. The more in tune we are with ourselves, and the healthier we feel within, the less other's opinions of us matter and the more we are able to serve ourselves and those around us from an authentic and genuine place.

I know I would rather feel grounded, happy and connected to the world around me than wanting to be right, blaming others or fighting to be heard. Wanting to be understood and getting caught up in what other people think is exhausting and never ending. Sometimes being right can deplete you. You have to ask yourself, is it worth it?

Whether it's the thoughts you think, the words you say or the environment you spend time in, imagine the impact it will have on your life when consciously creating coherence becomes habitual and becomes your normal response to daily challenges.

Chapter 23

HAVING AN OPEN HEART

Having an open heart is a universal concept taught by many spiritual traditions as well as some of the most inspiring teachers and thought leaders on the planet. I had heard this phrase many times and could conceptualize it, but I had a hard time feeling it.

Ultimately, we all want to feel love. Unfortunately, when the hormones of stress are rampant, there are literally thousands of chemical reactions going on in the brain and body that make it hard to *feel the love*.

When I was overloaded with stress, one of the ironies was how incoherent it felt to watch other people act lovingly towards each other.

When your heart is closed, you are in a state of separation and divisiveness. It's hard to feel positive about people who are connecting beautifully to one another.

There were many times I watched people who appeared happy and loving, and I just couldn't believe it was genuine. When I experienced anxiety over long periods of time, I found it challenging to be truly present and loving towards someone else. Watching people who were authentically happy became depleting for me and elicited emotions such as jealousy and resentment.

Depleting emotions tend to spiral unnecessarily. I felt guilty that I didn't feel happy for someone who bought their dream home, when I wanted mine. How could I be happy for someone else who had the opportunity to travel the world, when I could not? How could I be happy with my career and reach my goals if I always felt like I was struggling financially?

Whether I was truly struggling or not was irrelevant here. You see, if my perception was that I was struggling, then that was the lens through which I saw my life.

As I explored different ways to heal, I began to consciously observe people who acted in genuinely loving ways. I started to focus on how they sustained an open heart. When you are around someone whose heart is truly open, it's palpable. They usually emit a calming energy that feels authentic and safe.

I always questioned whether someone suffering with anxiety could create an open heart. If I wasn't creating the chemicals of love, happiness and joy all day, how could I? For the most part, all I ever created were the chemicals of stress. Could I achieve an open heart too? I felt terrible anxiety so often that trying to feel anything else in my heart didn't seem possible.

My perceptions started to change when I stopped looking at *getting rid of anxiety* as a destination and an end goal. Instead of figuring out why I was anxious, I focused on raising my vibration, drinking more water, eating something healthy or doing anything to change my physiological state. I wanted to have as many tools and options as I could to interrupt my negative patterns and reset my natural rhythm and emotional balance.

In the summer of 2019, my wife and I travelled to Portland, Oregon, and attended our third weeklong event with Dr. Joe Dispenza. My pattern at the beginning of the week was similar to the other events. I experienced a lot of self-judgment and a deep desire to fit in. There were some underlying emotions and fundamental doubts that continued to show up. After 30 years of working towards reduced anxiety and increased happiness, I still wasn't sure I could experience a genuine emotion or feel true happiness for other people.

As the week progressed, I found a better rhythm and eventually began to interact with others in a more joyful way. At some point in the middle of the week, I realized I was more interested in hearing people's stories and less interested in getting their approval. I was feeling less of a victim and more in control of my behavior. I even found myself taking part in the dancing which occurred after all the breaks. There was a palpable shift, and I felt more comfortable talking and interacting with all the different groups of people we had met. After several days of being in a room with over a thousand people consciously sharing love, I felt the impact in my heart.

During the last three days of a weeklong retreat with Dr. Joe, there are group healing sessions called Coherence Healings. I would say that amongst all those attending, roughly a quarter of participants are given the opportunity to receive a healing ('healee'). The remaining attendees are all participants ('healers') in the group healing experience.

Healing circles usually consist of nine people – eight people are 'the healers' who create a circle also known as 'the cage,' and the ninth enters the cage and is the recipient of the healing.

In preparation for these healings, Dr. Joe and his team promote *group coherence* through a meditation which guides participants to become heart-centered. A group trance is achieved with the use of beautiful video images depicting sacred geometry inside of a kaleidoscope. Imagine hundreds of people, heart-centered, in the same room!

After the meditation, participants are guided to build *coherence through movement* as they walk around the room to the rhythm of the music. It is such a unique and profound experience.

As the main group prepares for the healing sessions, the 'healees' are in a separate room with Dr. Joe as he guides them through a heart-centered meditation, encouraging them to receive the energy that will come their way. They are encouraged to surrender to the experience, to allow themselves to let go of old habits and to open their hearts to all that comes their way. Upon completion of the meditation, volunteers guide each 'healee' randomly to a heart-centered group of eight.

Aviva and I were fortunate to have the experience of being 'healers' in various groups of eight. On separate occasions, we each experienced the gift of being a 'healee.'

It would not be an exaggeration to say that as a 'healer,' I witnessed energetic shifts and healings that changed my perception of the world forever. I spoke with many people after their experience who told me of instant healings or dramatic recoveries over short periods of time. Some were almost instantaneous recoveries from strokes, asthma, depression, neurological disorders and even cancer. We literally witnessed miracles!

During the last day of our week in Portland, I was very fortunate to be chosen as a *healee*. The coherence healing lasted about thirty minutes, but it took some additional time for me to process the experience and come back to the present moment. To say I had a *heart opening* is an understatement! I felt sensations in my body and an inspiration for life that I had forgotten about. I felt that the *only* way to accurately explain my experience was to say that my *heart was open*.

When I finally looked around the room, other than slight confusion, I felt joy. I was excited to speak with people that only a few days ago had triggered a sense of insecurity in me. As I processed my experience, I eagerly wanted to hear other's experiences and share mine. I had a few heartfelt conversations, gave some hugs and told people I loved them.

I realized how genuine it all felt. I wasn't faking it; I felt it! There was no sense of jealousy, guilt or insecurity *and* there was no anxiety! I wasn't trying to *appear* like a loving person; I actually felt *loving* towards others!

The great thing about feeling your heart open is that the lens through which you view the world also changes and it becomes much easier to perceive possibility, gratitude and hope. When your heart is open, it feels natural to connect to yourself and others.

Chapter 24

TAKING ACTION

Daily Dream Life Schedule (DDLS)

Manifesting your *dream life* becomes a realistic goal when you put in the time to become clear on what that life looks like. By going through the *Coherence Revolution* process, you have the opportunity to explore and assess each aspect of your life and to deeply understand ways in which you can increase coherence and have conscious control over your emotional landscape.

The *Coherence Revolution* is meant to be a playful self-exploration that you can engage in as many times and as often as you'd like. The methods and situations you focus on to create coherence may often change. The more adaptable and aware you are of depleting situations, the more effectively you will be able to counteract them with renewed and uplifting emotional responses.

Once you have determined all of the elements you would like to include in your *dream life*, you are left with the most practical step of all – fitting it all in and making the time to follow through. Your goal may be to meditate, exercise, read, do yoga, spend time with friends, write in your journal or any other of an infinite number of possibilities. Finding a time that works for you is crucial. Everything usually sounds great until you try and implement your plan and realize you'll need 28 hours per day to live the life you've chosen.

Creating a DDLS is a process that helps you plan and make time for your dream life. When it is finished, it will provide the time for everything you choose and prioritize to be a part of your day. The chances of accomplishing your goals are greatly increased when you give yourself enough time to do so.

The first step is to decide when you would like to start and end your day. That sets the playing field, and defines how much time you have to work with. All of your non-negotiable commitments should be scheduled first, including your commuting time, specific hours of work, family responsibilities and meals.

Next, schedule time for your lifestyle and self-care. This may include such things as exercise, meditation, reading, watching a movie, writing, hobbies, social time and romance.

The last type of activities to be scheduled should always be the things that drain or deplete us that extra little bit, such as daily chores, shopping or laundry.

Most people plan their day on the fly and spend the majority of their time doing chores and the small unimportant things which leaves very little time for the things in life that contribute the most to health, happiness and contentment.

I have found that some people resist the idea of scheduling their life because they feel it will limit them and feel too controlled. I argue exactly the opposite. It is completely freeing to know that you have made time for and prioritized everything you would like to be a part of your life. Is it important to follow your schedule 100%? No!

This is a flexible template, and it's meant to support your ability to reach your goals and implement effective self-care. It is not meant to increase your responsibilities or be another unwanted stressor.

I have used a DDLS for many years, and I review and revise it a few times per year. The process of creating and following it as diligently as possible ensures that I am in the process of increasing coherence whenever possible.

The final step is perhaps the most important. As I discussed earlier, in many circumstances, it's less about what you're doing and more about what you are feeling. When you review your DDLS, spend a few moments identifying the types of emotions you would like to feel at specific times and parts of your day.

By identifying the emotions you would like to feel, you will have the opportunity to practice them. Additionally, by using your knowledge of nature and your senses on your emotional response, you can create environments that help facilitate the emotions you've chosen.

If you would like to feel an energized renewed emotion in the morning before work but a more tranquil emotion after work, are there different essential oils to help facilitate that? Are there images you would like to frame and display in a strategic area? Are there specific sounds or types of music that will help induce specific emotional responses? Which foods energize you and what would you eat when you want some comfort food? Is it possible for you to take a walk on a nature trail rather than a busy neighborhood street?

Explore as many options as you would like. Have fun with this step. Discover what works for you and be open and ready to adapt whenever it's necessary or simply because you'd like to try something new.

Rest and repair: travel vs. vacation

When designing your dream life, it's important to include time to rest and repair. Both your body and mind need time to unwind and recharge.

Although this can be accomplished in many ways, it is important to be aware of what you would like to achieve from your time off.

The saying, 'Wherever you go, there you are,' is never more appropriate than when discussing your valuable and cherished time off. Do you need down time or social time? Are you looking for adventure or to be catered to?

I have always distinguished between traveling and vacationing because to me, they are not the same thing. Travel, to me, has an exploratory aspect to it. It's about seeing something new, doing something different or having the opportunity to be creative in some way. Traveling always involves the sense of adventure. Although, for the sake of this discussion, travelling doesn't usually involve relaxation when you are engaged in an adventurous experience that inspires you. It is still a renewing experience that will result in feeling more rested and energized.

When I travel, one of my goals is to spend as much time doing activities where I experience being *in the zone*. I seek out activities that inspire me and stimulate a sense of curiosity. Memories of glacier climbing in Austria, shark diving in the Bahamas or skydiving in New Zealand are vivid and palpable. For many people, including myself at times, adventure may also be about tasting new foods, exploring different sites and encountering different cultures. However, adventure reveals itself in our lives; explorations awaken and invigorate the mind and the heart.

Vacationing, to me, is about rest. When I vacation, I want dependability. I want to know that my needs will be met and that the environment will help facilitate the healing and recovery my body desires. Vacationing is also about spending time in a relaxed, coherent state. It's restorative and it's a time that encourages renewal. Whether it's a short trip to the cottage, an all-inclusive resort, a weekend getaway or a staycation, it's an opportunity to rest, relax, laugh, love and reset.

Ultimately, whether you call it vacation, travelling or taking some time for yourself, it's just semantics. The important part is being conscious of what your needs are and planning your time accordingly.

The question is, do you have to go anywhere to get the renewal and recharging you are looking for? How many times have you fantasized about an upcoming trip only to find yourself on the trip feeling the same emotions as you did at home?

When you plan the trip, what you are really paying for and consciously planning for is the emotional state you want to achieve. It's less about the things you do and more about the emotions you feel during the time you're away as well as when you return.

This is another great example of how to use the power of creating coherence between your heart and brain by practicing different emotional states. Once you've decided on the type of vacation or trip you'd like to plan, you can identify the emotions you'd like to feel during that time and literally start practicing. As soon as you begin to practice the type of renewing emotions you'd like to feel while on holidays, you will start to reap the benefits. The irony is that you won't *need* the time away as much because you will be consciously renewing your own energy. Instead of acting out of desperation or lack, you will begin to make decisions based on what will truly satisfy your soul.

My process

Since the COVID-19 pandemic dominated the period when I was writing this book, I saw the value of going through the process again, playing out in real time. Could I show up as my best self?

The moment my chiropractic practice was shut down and I realized I was entering an even more uncertain period of time, I made a conscious decision to practice and start living as the person I wanted to be in that situation. Now granted, it was much easier to be the best me, at least with respect to devoting the time, because I simply had the time to do what was necessary while so many aspects of the external world were being closed, cancelled or unavailable.

There were definitely people who perceived the situation differently than I did because they believed it was much harder to be their best self during the pandemic due to the enormous amount of stress they experienced.

If that was your perspective, then you may have found yourself eating more, exercising and moving less, having very little motivation to be proactive and most likely feeling more irritable than you're used to.

I, fortunately, was the opposite. Although I knew it was perhaps the beginning of one of the most stressful periods of my life, I wasn't planning on watching my own tragedy unfold. Many of my past triggers were being tested. Thoughts of money, long-term security and my career were swirling around in my head. I had no idea how long the shutdown would last but I could hear my intuitive voice clearly saying, 'If I can't work, then I need to do something to make sure this time isn't wasted!'

During the first few days of the lockdown, I spent time grounding myself and gaining coherence so I could get clear on how I wanted to approach the circumstances I was stuck in. Once I had a couple of days to ground myself and raise my vibration, I felt more at peace with what was happening and was ready to make a plan.

What it boiled down to was being able to perceive my circumstances as a unique opportunity. I never wanted to look back and say I could have used the time better or even worse, let the stress of the situation affect my health and cause me suffering. I proceeded to look at my goals and think about what I wanted to accomplish both personally and professionally. I created a realistic DDLS that allowed me to feel I had covered all of my bases and scheduled time for everything that was important to me.

By following the basic outline of my DDLS, I gave myself permission to be in the moment. When I was working, I didn't have to worry about doing personal chores because I knew I made the time for that. When I spent time connecting with others or exercising or meditating, I was able to be more present because I knew that I was exactly where I chose to be.

In the past, I always felt rushed and in a hurry, whether it was warranted or not. Completing and implementing a DDLS has given me freedom as it allows me to feel like I have enough time for everything I've prioritized in my life.

During the shutdown, I started to take my time with everything. I didn't rush through any aspect of my schedule. Whether it was walking the dog, making a meal, writing or taking a shower, I practiced consciously, taking the extra minute or two to complete something properly and without stress. I reinforced that I could slow down and I still accomplished it all. I had plenty of time scheduled to accommodate all of my priorities. The schedule honored my need for periods of flexibility as well as structured time built in for self-care, my career and personal obligations.

Using this process helped me identify the best time of day for my version of a *Power Hour* that ranged anywhere between 30 – 90 minutes. Although the amount of time varied and the exact time of day changed, the time usually included meditation, breathwork, yoga and some form of vigorous exercise followed by a cold shower.

———————

Power hour is designated time, traditionally an hour, set aside every day, to either help you attain a goal or get things done. It is a time to ignore distractions and negative self-talk, take a break from technology and social media, avoid conversations and get laser focused on the outcome you would like to achieve.

———————

I found that by committing to this process, I attained a level of coherence that elevated my mood and positively impacted my entire day. After only a few weeks, I noticed that my ability to create and sustain coherence was improving, and I started to feel less erratic in my behavior and my thinking process.

Although I recommend you make a commitment to yourself to follow your DDLS, I also want to emphasize strongly that it is important to be flexible and give yourself plenty of options in your plan.

In my life, as long as I know I have scheduled enough time for everything that is important to me, I give myself the freedom to move things around or split the time in a way that makes sense for that day.

Many years ago, one of my mentors introduced a premise to me that has stuck with me to this day. 'If you underachieve on a daily basis, you will overachieve in life.'

He let me sit in my confusion at that concept for a moment and then explained further. Most people simply overwhelm themselves every day. As a society, we look up to people who are busy and seem to accomplish an enormous amount in their life. There is enormous pressure to *do more*. However, when your proverbial glass is completely full, there is no room for anything else to be added. When you overwhelm yourself with chores, work, socializing and even self-care, there is no room for regeneration, repair and ultimately, growth. If your goal is to increase the amount of energy, creativity and resilience you have, then one of the ways to do that is to assess your to-do list every day and consciously make a choice to reduce it by 10 – 15%. If you assess that something doesn't have to be done or can easily be done another time, then eliminate it from your day. Do a little bit less. When you end your day feeling like you were on top of everything, the next day doesn't feel nearly as intimidating either. Instead of overwhelming pressure, you will create the process of consistent growth.

In other words, you will overachieve in life when you consistently follow your process of underachieving tomorrow.

Creating the *Coherence Revolution* has inspired me and changed the course of my life. Committing to the process of creating coherence and choosing my emotional state has helped me perceive my life in new and exciting ways. The circumstances haven't changed. I've changed.

Doing and implementing the work

Anyone who has ever seen a therapist, taken a course or read a book will inevitably have gotten the message that to heal, you have to *do the work.*

What does *doing the work* actually mean?

Originally, for me, it meant being committed enough to the process of healing that it resulted in the elimination of my suffering and a complete resolution of the problem. It meant doing whatever it took, to go *all in* and fully commit to whatever method I was exploring at the time.

In most cases though, especially if you've hit rock bottom or are desperate for relief, it isn't a question of being committed. You'll most likely have no problem with that. It's about creating the most optimal process that allows you to live an authentic, heart-centered life. Remember, it's always about the process. If you stay committed to the process, positive results are the byproduct.

By the time I stopped searching for the cure to anxiety, I had plenty of options when it came to healthy habits, rituals, therapists, courses, books and technologies. I didn't want to miss out on anything. I always feared that if I didn't do it all, then I wouldn't get better, so I did a little bit of everything.

It took many years of trial and error before I was able to create and implement the successful systems I now use in my life. One of the most challenging aspects for me was slowing down and being mindful enough that I got the benefit from all the habits and processes I had implemented.

Although I found it hard to implement some of the new tools during episodes of severe anxiety, during periods of relatively low anxiety, I began to see some results from my efforts and felt a sense of satisfaction that I was setting myself up for success. I may not have been as *in the moment* as I would have liked, but I felt a sense of pride knowing that I made a conscious choice to gain coherence by practicing even a few minutes of yoga, writing in my gratitude journal, practicing HeartMath or meditating for a few minutes.

As I refined the strategies that worked for me, I had to consciously slow down. It became apparent that I was more focused on how many things I did rather than making sure I engaged in whatever I did optimally to maximize the benefits. All the healing modalities and good habits I attempted to implement just became things I could check off my list. I did my exercise, my meditation, my affirmations, HeartMath. Check, check, check, check.

I can still hear the voice in my head that echoed during those times. *Damn, I've used all of my tools and I still feel anxiety. Now what?*

Over the last two years the real meaning, or perhaps the deeper meaning of *doing the work,* has evolved significantly. *Doing the work* now refers to the process I've created in my life. It's about maximizing the amount of time I spend consciously creating renewed emotional states. Following the process *is* doing the work.

Once the process of creating coherence and changing unhelpful neurological programs becomes a primary daily focus, you begin to feel like you have more control over your future. You start to believe that you can manifest the life you want by practicing it.

Contrary to most things, creating coherence is not necessarily about achieving specific results. In other words, if you don't receive the results you want in the time frame anticipated, does it mean that creating coherence isn't valuable or doesn't work? Of course not.

Being in coherence does not mean that you will never face rejection, challenges or adversity. However, it will allow you to process and deal with negative outcomes a lot easier. If you make the effort to gain coherence during stressful events such as the death of a loved one, going through a divorce or getting fired from your job, you may still experience extreme stress; but you will have much more resilience. You will be able to think more clearly and make better decisions.

In each moment, it is always helpful to ask yourself how you can create more coherence. *Doing the work* means that all the healing modalities you use complement each other. It means that all of your financial decisions and purchases are in coherence with your goals. It means the way you earn money is coherent with your value system. It means that the people you choose to be around renew you rather than deplete you. It means the clothes you wear feel good on your body and it also means you like what you see when you look in the mirror. *Doing the work* means you are conscious of the words you use in every conversation. It means eating food that nourishes your body and making sure you are always hydrated. *Doing the work* means having a clear understanding of what you will and will not accept in your life. *Doing the work* means you see your own worth.

Will this work for you?

One of the most critical factors involved in achieving the results you are looking for is your belief that you will be successful. If you are wondering whether the *Coherence Revolution* will work for you, the answer is *yes!* The amount of time it will take may vary, but everyone can add coherence to their lives and learn how to consciously practice the emotions of their dream life.

This process is specifically designed without an end. It is a process that can be adapted and revised throughout your life. *Doing the work* is living the life you've created consciously.

Will you heal from disease? Repair a relationship? Rehabilitate an injury? It's possible. Things that have been deemed impossible occur all the time. Many people are given death sentences, yet they live. I've sat beside people who have healed from cancer, multiple sclerosis, paralysis from a stroke, colitis, allergies and dozens of other conditions. In the quantum world, research on the concepts of time, space and matter have given us new ways of understanding healing.

The intention of going through the *Coherence Revolution* is for you to gain awareness, and to gain conscious emotional control so you can create new possibilities for your future. When true healing occurs, it's not from attempting to treat the disease process, the damaged area or any specific issue at all. Healing occurs because when you experience a high degree of coherence in your brain and body, you change at a cellular level. Your energy changes, your emotions change and your symptoms change. You can change all the way down to your genetic code. When the emotions of your dream life become habitual, you will become a new person and it is entirely possible that your *new self* will not suffer with the same health conditions as your *old self* did.

Every time you resist the urge to fall back into old, hardwired programs and instead create a little more coherence, you're impacting your future. Remember, it's not the circumstances in your life that determine your happiness; it's your perception of them.

As you go through this process, it's important to continually reassess your goals and set your intentions. The easier it becomes to consciously evoke specific emotions, the more change you will perceive in your life.

Remember, creating real change in your hardwired programs will take a greater emotional response and more energy than the existing pattern, or nothing will happen.

Creating and sustaining behavioral and neurophysiological changes require a sincere effort.

Creating significant change in any of the habits or emotional responses that are preventing you from reaching your true potential will take your best effort and a willingness to go beyond what you have done in the past. It may not always make others happy and it may feel uncomfortable.

It will take time and persistence.

How much time?

Well, that depends on you, your soul, your journey. I have witnessed and been present for profound healings that were instantaneous.

I also know that some patterns are so intricately hardwired in your brain that they become a recurring pattern in your life.

My advice is always to do the work, stay in the present and try not to focus on how long things will take. Some things can change overnight while others, especially areas of deep trauma, may take many years for the full release.

Create your process and then live your process. Focus on being your best self in the present moment.

With the love and support from all of us at *Coherence Revolution*, you have a community of people who share the same goals and are implementing the same changes as you. We're all here to support each other on our quest to live our best lives.

That sounds like a revolution to me.

APPENDIX

Additional Resources

More influential books and programs

As I wrote this book, I wanted to ensure every concept resonated with me. I had learned so many interesting and life-changing skills that I wanted to make sure I didn't forget to include anything. I literally reviewed every book I've read that impacted and inspired me in some way.

I spent some time re-reading all the pages that I had originally folded in the upper corner as a reminder to review it later. I frequently used that method while reading, assuming that I would revisit the most impactful concepts. The funny part is, I never did. Until now. And talk about coherence! As I reviewed and looked through the books, it amazed me that the concepts I saved to review were all similar and on point with what I was trying to accomplish. Coincidence? Nope. *Coherence.*

Adam the DreamHealer

These are a series of books about Adam, who has an incredible ability to utilize energy for healing purposes. When I attended his workshop, he read the entire aura of everyone in the room. There were hundreds of people and I could actually see layers of colourful light that were shifting and intensifying all around us.

I enjoyed reading this series of books and I found Adam's story fascinating. He had the same type of ability as Dr. Eric Pearle did to access and manipulate different frequencies of energy. The more I studied and saw what others were capable of doing, the more motivated I was to continue learning and pushing my own boundaries.

The Diamond Cutter

The Diamond Cutter was based on a true story of a man who implemented Buddhist principles in a business he operated in the New York diamond industry. This book successfully highlights Buddhist principles that can be used for business management rather than the more Western-based approaches. Some of the suggestions, especially how to relate to his employees, seemed counterintuitive at first. Once I tried them myself, they felt more congruent and I got the results I was looking for.

As I've gone through the process of writing and looking at the world from a coherent versus incoherent state, I have gained a better understanding of many of the concepts I've learned over the last 25 years. One of the aspects I really appreciate about this book, and about Buddhism, is that it helps to clarify the idea of being in flow or in sync with something or someone else.

For example, if you are an employer trying to train your employees on protocols that are essential for a profitable business, forcing compliance is not a good strategy. It is extremely unlikely you will be successful if you try to reprimand people into learning something new. Financial success is rarely the result of a hostile dynamic.

By using the specific Buddhist principles taught in *The Diamond Cutter*, your actions and communications with people could be approached from a new perspective that helps facilitate more congruent energy and *social coherence*. The intention is to create an environment where everyone will thrive.

The Sedona Method

One of the first techniques that helped me become more mindful and aware of my thoughts was *The Sedona Method*. This system helps analyze words, statements and beliefs that race through your mind. It teaches you to be conscious of your word choice and how to replace some of the unwanted statements you use when talking with yourself.

The Sedona Method is a great way to start creating more coherence between your conscious and your subconscious beliefs because every time you question a thought or belief you have the opportunity to reprogram your mind.

One of the big takeaways from *The Sedona Method* for me was asking myself the following question: do you want to let go of your problem, or do you want to understand why?

Sometimes letting go means letting go of needing to know why. You are always allowed to entertain any emotional state or thought process you choose. It is not about stopping you from going through an emotion. When you feel stuck, ask yourself, 'Is feeling a strong negative emotion beneficial for me in this moment?'

Fractal Time

Gregg Braden has written some fascinating books, and *Fractal Time* was no exception. One concept that helped me see life through a different lens was when he talked about '*the conditions for something to occur*.' In other words, sometimes an event will occur and sometimes it won't, even if the *conditions to occur* are present. For example, the conditions to play golf are perfect outside but that doesn't necessarily mean you will play golf. From a global perspective, the conditions for war might be present but it doesn't mean it will occur. Human choice exists, which means it can be avoided if both parties want to find a resolution.

From a coherence perspective, a good example would involve the state of mind you are in. Meditating and practicing breathwork both relax your mind and body and increase your resilience. They are powerful habits used to create the proper conditions in your mind to cope with a stressful event but it doesn't mean there will actually be a stressful event. It is healthy for your brain to be in a state of mind capable of handling a stressful event regardless if it occurs.

Gregg also has a way of explaining and introducing complicated concepts, such as *global coherence* and our relationship to time and space, in easily understandable and accessible ways.

Gregg Braden joins Dr. Bruce Lipton and Dr. Joe Dispenza as thought leaders and guides for people exploring the new fields of science including quantum physics and epigenetics.

Centerpointe

I started using Centerpointe technology in the early 2000s. It was the first modality I used to directly influence the way my brain functioned. The program consisted of a series of audio recordings that used specific frequencies and binaural beat technology. Each session was like a workout for the brain. The purpose of the program was to gradually retrain and reprogram the brain. With consistent use, the technology helps the brain reduce the intensity and amount of stressful brain wave patterns and increases the brain waves which facilitate relaxation and healing.

The recordings were a passive experience. I didn't have to do anything except lay back and listen. There were several main challenge levels and each one consisted of 8-10 recordings. It was my understanding that each successive level got more difficult.

I didn't really know how to gauge if I was having success, but if I progressed up a level too quickly, I'd feel a strange, intense pressure in my head as I lay there. Every time it happened, I was lying on my back in a meditative state, when suddenly I'd feel very uncomfortable. It wasn't pain, or loud noise, or nausea or any sensation I could explain. I just wanted to take the earphones off my head if it got too intense. When I took my time at each level, I had a much easier time adapting.

Over the course of many months, I progressed several levels. I enjoyed the meditations but during that period of time, I discovered so many new and hopeful options to try that I eventually moved on. As I look back and put context to my journey, I am grateful for my experience with the Centerpointe technology and view it as the precursor to the BrainTap technology I found years later.

The Secret

The Secret is both a book and movie. At the time of its release, it was significant because it was the biggest project of its kind and involved many of the thought leaders in the self-help, alternative health and quantum energy fields.

The Secret became a huge phenomenon not only because it had inspiring authors and speakers, but also because they were able to create a viral marketing campaign which created a lot of buzz around The Secret and its key concept, the law of attraction.

Over the years, there has been some criticism of *The Secret* because of what was seen as a critical omission. There was very little discussion about the *emotional retraining* that is needed to properly initiate the law of attraction. In my opinion, *The Secret* didn't emphasize the necessity of a strong positive emotional response in conjunction with the visualization to fuel the attraction.

The effectiveness of the law of attraction is directly connected to the intensity of the emotion attached to the goal.

The Hidden Messages in Water

It is incredibly inspiring to view all the beautiful images and crystal formations studied by Dr. Emoto. To me, his work feels like it's on the verge of explaining some of life's mysteries. You can certainly infer a lot about humanity.

Reading through the volumes of Dr. Emoto's work provides an eye-opening look at how words affect all of us at a cellular level. It is easy to conclude that the words we use and the thoughts we think towards ourselves and others can and will drastically affect our health as well as the health of those around us.

5 Love Languages

Although the term is not used in the book, I believe that the concept of *communication coherence* is the true essence of *5 Love Languages*. While we can say that humans crave love, the way in which each person defines, gives and receives love can vary greatly. In the *5 Love Languages*, the author, Gary Chapman, explores the different communication styles and methods used to give and receive love.

After reading the book, I had a much deeper understanding of how people resonate with and are affected differently by specific types of physical actions, tones of voice, choice of words and emotional responses.

It is crucial, when creating a coherent relationship, to understand your partner's love language and to ensure that your communication is renewing for both of you.

Secrets of the Millionaire Mind

Secrets of the Millionaire Mind was one of the first books I read on the subject of subconscious belief patterns. I found it engaging and I resonated with the idea of resetting financial subconscious beliefs. The book was filled with practical exercises and assignments. If I was willing to be conscious and proactive, I could ensure I had all the belief systems necessary to achieve financial success.

When I bought the book, I was lucky enough to also receive an invitation to attend a two-day seminar on developing a healthy financial belief system. By combining the knowledge from the book with the live experience, I was able to create a financial blueprint that was coherent with my life.

Happy for No Reason

Happy for No Reason provides various ways to create more happiness in your life. I just simply like this book.

It's a book that I've revisited and reviewed many times. Each time, my perception and interpretation of the material has evolved. The entire book is focused on providing the reader with ways to create renewing emotions and inevitably increased coherence.

The concept of *practicing happiness* was introduced to me in this book. It became a fundamental principle in my life because it just made sense to me that rather than searching for happiness, I would begin to practice happiness.

Happiness can become an unconscious habit when the emotion

becomes hardwired and the brain habitually creates *happy chemicals*, independent of what is happening in your life.

Creating a new set point for happiness is all about training and repetition. While this practice can be tedious at times and takes consistent effort, it is definitely worthwhile. *Happy for No Reason* offers many tools to help with this process.

GLOSSARY OF IMPORTANT TERMS AND CONCEPTS

Allostatic Load

Allostatic load refers to the long-term effects of continued exposure to chronic stress on the body. Colloquially, it is often referred to as 'wear and tear.' Allostatic load can be increased due to dysfunctional coping mechanisms such as a repeated failure to habituate to common stressors and an inadequate response from one or more bodily responses that leads to hyperactivity in other bodily responses to stress.

The term allostatic load was coined by researchers Bruce S. McEwen and Elliot Stellar in 1993. (Source: https://www.hrzone.com/hr-glossary/what-isallostatic-load)

Amygdala

The amygdala is an emotional processing center in our brain that contains snapshots of emotional memories. It's also a pattern-matching system that scans your brain for familiarity so you can respond to a situation in the same manner you did last time. For example, if you felt feelings of anxiety, anger or sadness as a result of a past event, the same emotions can be triggered if a similar situation presents itself. Eventually, the response can become conditioned to occur even before you've had time to think about whether it is an appropriate response or not.

Autonomic Nervous System (ANS)

The autonomic nervous system is the part of the nervous system responsible for control of the bodily functions not consciously directed, such as breathing, the heartbeat and digestive processes. The sympathetic nervous system and the parasympathetic nervous system constitute the autonomic nervous system. The ANS is a highly intelligent system guiding 90% of the body's processes. It is fair to call it the *subconscious mind*, as it intelligently manages a complex array of processes without our *conscious mind* needing to be involved. Patterns we talk about as coming from 'the subconscious' have their physiological anchor in the autonomic nervous system. When we learn to bring balance within the autonomic nervous system and release old trauma, we are transforming and releasing long-held patterns in our subconscious, not just changing our physiology.

Sympathetic nervous system. A part of the nervous system that serves to accelerate the heart rate, constrict blood vessels and raise blood pressure.

The sympathetic nervous system directs the body's rapid involuntary response to dangerous or stressful situations. A flash flood of hormones boosts the body's alertness and heart rate, sending extra blood to the muscles.

Parasympathetic nervous system. The parasympathetic nervous system is sometimes called the rest-and-digest system. It conserves energy as it slows the heart rate, increases intestinal and gland activity and relaxes sphincter muscles in the gastrointestinal tract.

Brain Wave Frequencies

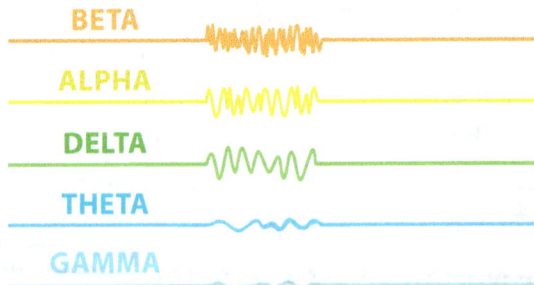

BETA

ALPHA

DELTA

THETA

GAMMA

Beta waves (12 to 38 Hz). Beta brain waves dominate our normal waking state of consciousness when attention is directed towards cognitive tasks and the outside world. Beta is a 'fast' activity, present when we are alert, attentive, engaged in problem solving, judgment, decision-making or focused mental activity. High beta wave frequencies are more predominant during periods of stress.

Alpha waves (8 to 12 Hz). Alpha brain waves are dominant during quietly flowing thoughts, and in some meditative states. Alpha is 'the power of now', being here, in the present. Alpha is the resting state for the *brain*. Alpha waves aid overall mental coordination, calmness, alertness, mind/body integration and learning.

Theta waves. Theta activity has a frequency of 3.5 to 7.5 Hz and is classed as 'slow' activity. It is seen in connection with creativity, intuition, daydreaming and fantasizing, and is a repository for memories, emotions and sensations. Theta waves are strong during internal focus, meditation, prayer and spiritual awareness.

Delta waves. Delta brain waves are slow, loud brainwaves (low frequency and deeply penetrating, like a drum beat). They are generated in deepest meditation and dreamless sleep. Delta waves suspend external awareness and are the source of empathy.

Gamma brain waves are the fastest brain waves produced inside your brain. Although they can be hard to measure accurately, they tend to measure above 35 Hz and can oscillate as fast as 100 Hz. Your brain tends to produce gamma waves when you're intensely focused or actively engaged in solving a problem. (Source: http://www.healthline.com)

Coherence

Coherence can be defined in several ways depending on the context of the situation. For some, it's a process of connecting with their spirit, higher power, universal source or God. For others, it's becoming consciously aware of the unified field, the quantum aspects to brain function and utilizing the power of nature to live their best life.

According to the HeartMath Institute, it's 'an optimal state in which the heart, mind and emotions are operating in-sync and are balanced.

Physiologically, the immune, hormonal and nervous systems function in a state of energetic coordination. Coherence is a scientific term that describes a highly efficient, health-promoting state associated with positive emotion and a high degree of mental and emotional stability. In other words, physiologically, there is heart alignment between your mental, emotional and physical system and you feel balanced and energized.'

Coherence is a scientific term that appropriately defines the *flow state,* or being *in the zone.*

Auditory coherence occurs when any sound or frequency stimulates or increases coherence in any aspect of your being and helps you access renewing emotional states.

Career coherence occurs when the job or career you choose inspires you, gives you purpose, easily funds your lifestyle and facilitates renewal of your emotional system.

Cellular coherence occurs when the cells of every system in your body vibrate in a synchronous frequency that produces optimal function and results in a healthy mind and body.

Coherent communication occurs when words, gestures, interactions, touch or body language stimulate or increase coherence in any aspect of your being and help you access renewing emotional states.

Digestive coherence is the optimal process that occurs as the body breaks down food into the most effective and efficient building blocks used to produce fuel and energy for the body.

Emotional coherence is the result of your ability to create a situationally appropriate emotional response that encourages a renewal of your emotional system rather than one of overwhelm.

Financial coherence occurs when your job / career or your investments result in enough wealth to create and manifest your financial desires. The financial stress you've experienced in the past can be released by developing an understanding and a belief that you will always have enough. Ultimately, *financial coherence* leads to financial freedom.

Global coherence is the optimal vibrational state of our planet as it relates to supporting all forms of life.

Kinesthetic coherence occurs when any physical movement, touch or sensory stimuli increases coherence in any aspect of your being and helps you access renewing emotional states.

Olfactory coherence occurs when any smell stimulates or increases coherence in any aspect of your being and helps you access renewing emotional states.

Social coherence occurs at a cellular level when the electromagnetic fields of different people resonate with each other. When there is harmony or resonance between human beings, an attraction or affinity towards each other is formed.

Subconscious coherence is the result of a healthy state of mind and body flowing out of subconscious beliefs that are congruent with your conscious belief system.

Taste coherence occurs when the taste of any ingestible substance stimulates or increases coherence in any aspect of your being and helps you access renewing emotional states.

Visual coherence occurs when any visual stimuli increases coherence in any aspect of your being and helps you access renewing emotional states.

Epigenetics

Epigenetics is an emerging field of science that studies how genetic traits are exhibited, altered or inhibited due to environmental factors to which we are all exposed. Several lifestyle and environmental factors have been identified that might modify epigenetic patterns, such as diet, obesity, physical activity, tobacco smoking, alcohol consumption, environmental pollutants, psychological stress and working on night shifts (Epigenetics – National Human Genome Research Institute).

Happy Chemicals

There are four primary chemicals that drive positive emotions.

- **Dopamine** is known as the reward chemical. It is released after completing a task, doing self-care, eating food and celebrating wins.

- **Serotonin** is known as the mood stabilizer. It is released during meditation, sun exposure, walking in nature, swimming and cycling.

- **Oxytocin** is known as the love hormone. It is released while playing with a dog or a baby, holding hands, hugging family and giving a compliment.

- **Endorphins** are released while laughing, using essential oils, watching a comedy, eating dark chocolate and doing exercise.

Neurological Interrupt

A *neurological interrupt* can be defined as any conscious or unconscious thought, action or behavior that occurs with enough intensity and emotion that it interrupts the unwanted hardwired pattern, changes your focus and reinforces your new desired response.

Schumann Resonance

'At any given moment, about 2,000 thunderstorms roll over Earth, producing some 50 flashes of lightning every second. Each lightning burst creates electromagnetic waves that begin to circle around Earth captured between Earth's surface and a boundary about 60 miles up. Some of the waves- if they have just the right wavelength- combine, increasing in strength, to create a repeating atmospheric heartbeat known as Schumann resonance.' (NASA)

Being out of sync with the Schumann resonance (Earth's heartbeat) can be depleting and can lead to health concerns such as anxiety, insomnia, illness and a suppressed immune system. Conversely, when we are in sync with the Earth's heartbeat, the body is able to heal and renew itself.

Stress

Stress is one of the largest contributors and determining factors in the development of disease and your ability to heal effectively. Your brain and nervous system can only adapt to and tolerate a limited amount of stress before losing efficiency and resilience. Accumulation of stress reduces your body's ability to cope with the stressors of daily life.

Types of Stress

Physical stress. The body requires movement and physical activity. The musculoskeletal and postural system is under constant physical strain from common forces such as gravity and ground reactive forces. The body thrives on positive physical stimulation called eustress. When the postural system becomes overwhelmed by chronic or acute physical stressors, it is termed de-stress (distress). Typical stressors include repetitive strain, sitting, sport injuries, car accidents, scoliosis, poor sleep position, flat feet, standing on hard floors, lifting/carrying.

Chemical stress. Chemical stress occurs when external substances place an added burden on the body. Chronic chemical stress is a large contributor to poor health. Some examples include processed food, drugs, alcohol, caffeine, medications, aspartame, nicotine and carbon dioxide.

Chemicals of stress. When stress triggers communication between the hypothalamus and the pituitary, the adrenal glands produce and release the stress hormones – epinephrine (also known as adrenaline), norepinephrine (noradrenaline) and cortisol.

Emotional stress. A state of emotional and mental strain resulting from your perception that a situation is challenging or overwhelming.

Electromagnetic stress. We may experience electromagnetic stress through our exposure to technology such as television, computer, tablet, phone, Bluetooth and many other devices which emit different electromagnetic fields. Electromagnetic frequencies (EMF) or electromagnetic radiation (EMR) emit from these devices and can disrupt normal cell function and contribute to poor health.

Special thank you to HeartMath for giving permission to use their images.

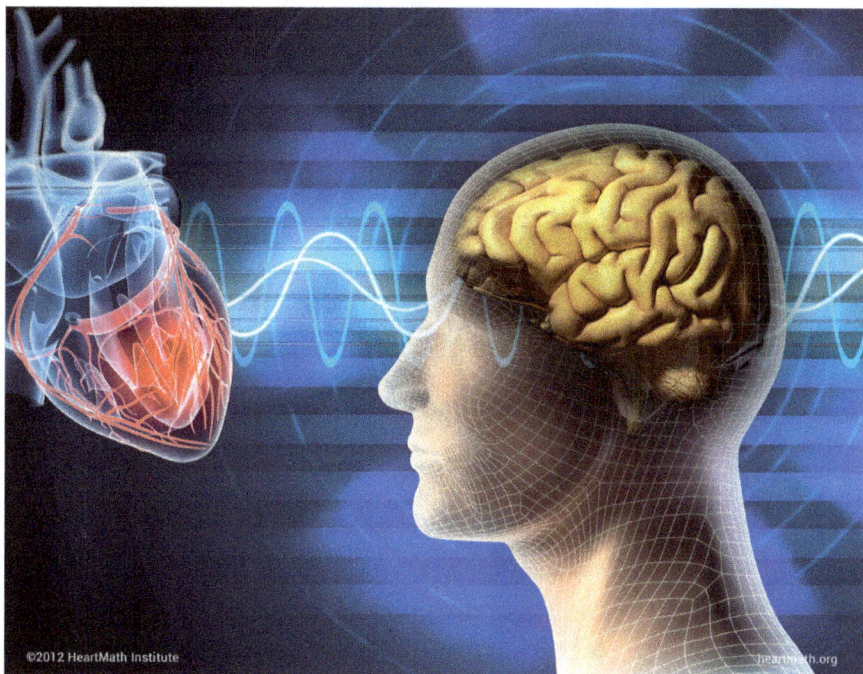

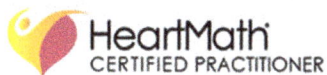

©2012 HeartMath Institute

heartmath.org

HeartMath
CERTIFIED PRACTITIONER

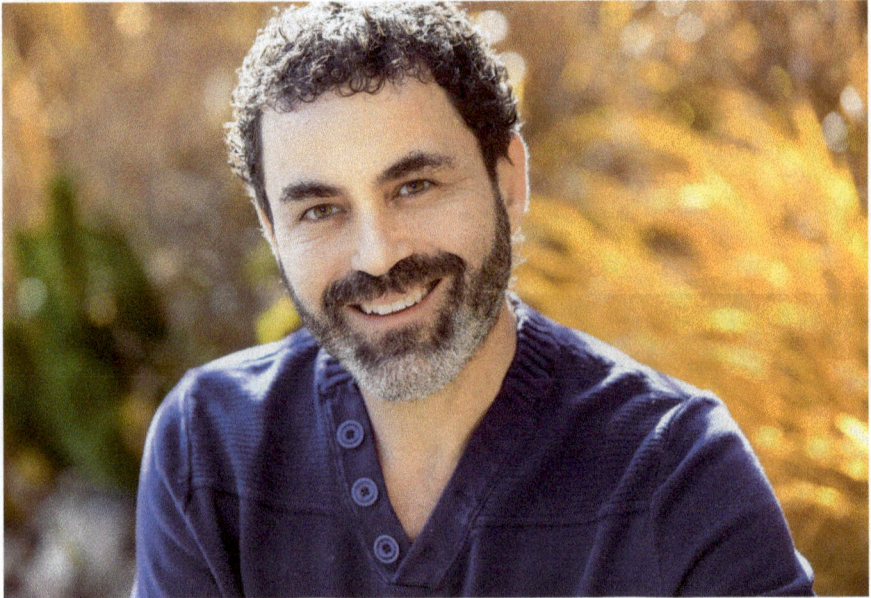

ABOUT THE AUTHOR

Dr. Mark Halpern is a Chiropractor, Author, Lecturer and Certified HeartMath Practitioner. He is also certified in additional healing modalities; PSYCH-K and Ho'oponopono. In both his personal and professional life, Dr. Mark has been drawn to methods that promote optimal health and healing of the brain, body and spirit.

Having found success navigating his own journey through stress and anxiety, Dr. Mark created the Coherence Revolution to share years of experience-based research on self-inquiry and personal growth.

Dr. Mark Halpern has been in practice since 1996. He is the founder and CEO of Coherence Revolution. He resides in Toronto, Canada, with his wife Aviva; two children, Jessica and Andrew and their fur baby, Gracie Rhythm.